SUE SCARFE

A Journey Through Dementia

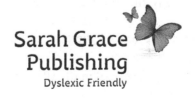

Sarah Grace
Publishing
Dyslexic Friendly

Copyright © Sue Scarfe 2024

First published 2024 by Sarah Grace Publishing,
an imprint of Malcolm Down Publishing Ltd
www.sarahgracepublishing.co.uk

28 27 26 25 24   7 6 5 4 3 2 1

The right of Sue Scarfe to be identified as the author of this
work has been asserted by her in accordance with the Copyright,
Designs and Patents Act 1988.

British Library Cataloguing in Publication Data
A catalogue record for this book is available from the British Library.

ISBN 978-1-915046-92-5

Unless otherwise indicated, Scripture quotations are taken from
the Holy Bible, New International Version (Anglicised edition)
Copyright ©1979, 1984, 2011 by Biblica. Used by permission of
Hodder & Stoughton Publishers, an Hachette UK company.
All rights reserved.

'NIV' is a registered trademark of Biblica.
UK trademark number 1448790.

Cover design by Esther Kotecha
Art direction by Sarah Grace

Typeface: The Grace Typeface® by 2K Denmark

Printed in the UK

Contents

Foreword

This is not a story, or a narrative. This is a truth. This is real. Its sadness is equalled only in its hope and faith. Throughout our time working together Sue and I have had, and continue to share, moments of joy, disagreement, anger, pain, elation and humour. Most of all, though, what will remain with me is the phrase that kept returning: "It was real."

Their marriage, their faith, their suffering, their experiences. They were all real. At first, I took this term at face value: they existed, they happened, they had a real-ness . . . so what? Then I began to see that this simple sentence encapsulated more than experience; it described a way of being that so beautifully depicts Sue, her life, her marriage, and her journey through dementia.

Being real is hard. It's ugly. It does not have any quick wins, can certainly be a struggle in the moment, and becomes a mammoth task over a lifetime. However, being real also offers a deeper intimacy into oneself, into relationships, into faith. To be real is to go beyond the imagination or fantasy. It is to harness the courage and strength to meet the reality in front of you with congruence, authenticity and a healthy dose of humour!

Whether being real comes easily as you deliver a course you love, or packaged more challengingly by hearing the news you fear the most, being real is the key to connection. It is the difference between hopping between islands to avoid the sea of despair, and finding a way to flow between them, integrating despair with love, joy and hope. Being real connects you to yourself, provides the basis for connecting to others and in turn the openness to receive the full spectrum of light, love and support from those around you.

It seems almost laughable now, but one very useful "therapeutic device" was provided not by me, but by the colourful leggings adorned by Sue. I could wax lyrical about the symbolism or latent and manifest meanings to be found in those patterns. However, this is not a book about leggings. It is about truth; it is about reality. The leggings were there, we were there, and we continue to be as real with each other as the leggings themselves.

Colin Houlihan
BA, PGDip, MSc, MBACP

Chapter 1

A Magical Belief

As a child I believed in Father Christmas, and I believed in God. In fact, I thought they were the same person. I loved Christmas with the tinsel and the excitement, and I also loved my Bible story book about Jesus calming the storm, about him healing all the people, about how much he loved me. It all seemed very straightforward and magical.

My whole family attended a small Methodist chapel where I felt special and loved every Sunday, especially as I saw my two grandmas and my uncles Dave and Ken who all made such a fuss of me. My uncle Dave, a vibrant man in his twenties, led Sunday school, making it fun but also real. He took me camping in the New Forest, to the zoo, sledging in the snow and on cycle rides. He loved God and seemed to know him personally. I believed what he taught so when he told us the story of God calling Samuel in the Bible, I expected to hear an audible voice calling me. When he told us stories of Jesus healing, I believed in Jesus the healer.

As I grew up I stopped believing in Father Christmas, but I still believed that, as a Christian, life would go well, and that God would wave his magic wand and make everything better.

God was not Father Christmas, though, giving out shiny gift-wrapped presents. Life was not a fairy tale with God as the rescuing prince that made all things go well without any troubles or problems. Jesus said, "In this world you will have trouble" (John 16:33). He also said, "Never will I leave you; never will I forsake you" (Hebrews 13:5).

This book is about my faith journey through the difficulties and questioning. It is about real life and a God who was with me through the troubles and heartache.

At the age of twelve I discovered that I could share the concerns of life with a God who cared about me. When I was struggling with difficulties at school, or when I thought my parents were being unfair, I climbed the apple tree at the bottom of the garden and talked to God about it. I felt his presence and I often heard him speaking to me deep within my heart. I realised that life could be hard, and I asked Jesus to come into my heart and to help me as I faced growing up.

Once at senior school, I discovered how much I enjoyed sports and gymnastics, and I decided to be a PE teacher. At the age of fifteen we had careers talks at school, but I was not interested as I was convinced that I knew what I wanted to do. On one occasion I was sitting in the school hall, not listening to a head teacher of a special school mumbling in a most uninteresting manner, when suddenly I experienced God's voice so clearly saying he wanted me to teach mentally handicapped children, the right term at the time for those with a severe learning disability. I walked out of that school hall in a daze, saying, "But I have never met a mentally handicapped child." A few weeks later I was given the opportunity to volunteer at a long-stay hospital for the mentally handicapped. I loved it and realised God knew me so well, so I excitedly applied for a teacher training course with a special needs specialty, and was accepted. I thoroughly enjoyed college and met like-minded people who all wanted to make life better for those with a disability. We were going to change the world for these children and ensure that they were not forgotten but would be loved and valued. I remember stating, "If someone with cognitive impairment is loved they could be happy and enjoy life, as long as they were not in physical pain." I was on a mission!

At the time in the 1970s, most mentally handicapped children resided in long-stay hospitals, in impersonal wards looked after by nursing staff. My first teaching job was in a school in the grounds of one of those hospitals. My class consisted of eight children who were all nonverbal, and I proceeded to put all I learned into practice.

Chapter 2

God, My Protector and Healer

Soon after starting my career, I met my first husband. I naively assumed that as we were both Christians our marriage would be successful. Even our church minister told us before the wedding that he usually gave marriage preparation classes, "But," he stated, "you two don't need that." He was so wrong. I still had magical thinking that God would wave his wand and all would be well. In fact, I had no idea how to navigate through the unknown territory of relationship.

We were both thrilled when soon after the wedding I became pregnant. I felt like a mother right from the start and knew that my child was such a gift from God.

A few weeks later, one Sunday I was helping at Sunday school when one of the children felt ill and spent the whole of the morning sitting on my lap. I didn't think anything of it and obviously told her mum when she came to pick her up. The next day the mum appeared at my door and told me that her daughter had German measles (rubella). I was mortified and very frightened as I knew how dangerous rubella was to an unborn child and I had not been vaccinated. The rubella vaccinations had only been offered to fourteen-year-old girls when I was sixteen, as they did not want to vaccinate us at sixteen because legally we could have sex and therefore we could be pregnant. Giving a rubella vaccination when pregnant would have devastating consequences. In my class of eight, two had disabilities caused by rubella. They were deaf or had partial hearing, had partial sight, were cognitively impaired and were unable to speak. They were both twelve years old and were from a West Indian background. There were many similar in the hospital as families had moved to England at a time when there was an outbreak of German measles, and many children were damaged in the womb. What an awful start to what they all thought was going to be a new beginning for them!

I went to the GP who told me that they would test me to see if I had antibodies. I was negative, which meant I was at risk of rubella. They would test me again in three weeks and if I had a positive response this time it would mean that I had contracted rubella, and even if I had no symptoms my baby would be affected. "Don't worry," explained the doctor, "we would give you a termination." I was livid. This was my child he was talking about! I wanted protection, not destruction for my baby. I thought he seemed very unfeeling.

The wait seemed interminable as I cried, and I prayed. I had always thought I would write a book and now I imagined that God was going to ask me to write a book about my own child. I did not want to write a book about bringing up a child damaged by rubella. I didn't want to test my belief that if a child was loved they could live a happy life, even with cognitive impairment, and then write a book about it.

God was gracious, though, and spoke lovingly to me. He told me to give him my child and to name her Lisa. In those days we had no idea what gender babies were until they were born, so I had no idea whether my baby would be a girl. But I looked up the meaning of the name Lisa. It means "Consecrated to God". I had no human means of protecting my child, so I placed her in God's hands. The next test was negative. Despite the very probable outcome after sitting with the young girl in Sunday school, my baby and I had not contracted rubella. Several months later, I had a beautiful healthy girl named Lisa.

I believe God protected Lisa. My faith soared and my childhood belief that God could do the impossible and could heal today was confirmed.

I loved being a mum and Lisa was followed eighteen months later by her brother, Geoffrey. I had not realised how hard and tiring it was bringing up a family. Richard, my husband, and I put a lot of energy into being there for our children. I am sure we made mistakes but somehow, they grew up into their teens knowing they were loved. Though we worked together as parents we were much less successful in our relationship with each other. I am not going to air our struggles but suffice to say our marriage broke down and we separated and later divorced. I felt such a failure and had so much guilt. As a Christian I had assumed that my marriage would not only last but would be stable and successful. My mental health suffered, and I sank into clinical depression.

I had always said that God loved everyone, including me, and I confidently taught this in Sunday school, demonstrated it in my teaching job and shared it with my children. Now, however, I felt I had failed, couldn't serve God and imagined I never would be able to again. I had nothing to give, and I realised that despite knowing God loved everyone unconditionally, I had also behaved as though I had earned his love by the things I did. My journey led me on a painful path of healing and restoration, but the consequences led me to really believe that God loved me, really loved me even though I had fallen badly. It was truly his unconditional love that I felt at my lowest point.

Chapter 3

Authentic Love

I gradually recovered and started out on a journey of growth. I realised I had so much to learn about myself, my feelings, my inadequacies and my relationships. Life was not as straightforward as I had come to believe. It was a painful process, but God was with me in the pain.

I started to talk with a friend, Adrian, with whom I could share honestly without pretence. We talked authentically for hours, and we soon realised we were in love.

As our relationship progressed, I started thinking of him as my soulmate. I felt so loved and accepted; he loved me as I was, the real me, and he encouraged me to be the person God made me to be and to be honest with my feelings. He saw me as a flower blossoming. We had a real relationship with its ups and downs and frustrations and arguments, but we always got through them. He never put me down, belittled me, abused me or demanded from me. He had great respect for me and, in fact, others too. I grew in confidence and although life was hard at times, I felt loved and supported.

Adrian was a counsellor who worked with people with a gambling addiction. He understood their issues and helped them through them. He also trained other counsellors and helpline staff, spoke at conferences, and often travelled internationally. I remember the time he was invited to speak at a conference in New Zealand. I went with him, and we were able to build a holiday around it. It was the start of an amazing time travelling together to parts of the world I never believed I would see. It was fantastic seeing God's creation – the glaciers of Alaska, the fjords of Norway, the Caribbean, the Rockies of Canada and much more.

We felt God's presence with us. We prayed together, real authentic prayers, speaking honestly with God. Adrian said he wanted to be with me, to marry me but also to work with me.

I was teaching men with learning disabilities, mental health issues and offending behaviour within an NHS medium-secure unit. I knew that God had a heart for the vulnerable, those who were on the margins of society, those who were hurting, those who had messed up. Together we wanted to reach out to the broken, the hurting and the hopeless. We wanted to bring God's love and healing and show them that there was hope, hope for all of us, whatever our past.

We felt that our mission was that of Isaiah 61:1-3:

> The Spirit of the Sovereign LORD is on me, because the LORD has anointed me to proclaim good news to the poor. He has sent me to bind

up the broken-hearted, to proclaim freedom for the captives and release from darkness for the prisoners, to proclaim the year of the LORD's favour and the day of vengeance of our God, to comfort all who mourn, and provide for those who grieve in Zion – to bestow on them a crown of beauty instead of ashes, the oil of joy instead of mourning, and a garment of praise instead of a spirit of despair. They will be called oaks of righteousness, a planting of the LORD for the display of his splendour.

We both knew God's healing for our brokenness, and we wanted to share this with others, to bring God's unconditional love to others who were in pain. We also wanted to commit ourselves to a loving marriage to each other. We knew that we needed God for both these things.

Adrian shared with me a verse from the Bible that he felt God gave him for our future. "A cord of three strands is not quickly broken" (Ecclesiastes 4:12). My engagement ring represented this, consisting of two small diamonds with a sapphire between them. We were joined together by God in the middle.

I was so happy, and I basked in the authentic love that I was experiencing. I could share everything with Adrian. We had fun, we had intimacy, we travelled, we had hope, our future looked bright. My children blessed our relationship and later our marriage. Both my children married and had their children, who became Adrian's grandchildren as well. He had never had his own children and he was so appreciative of being welcomed into my family.

Other people could see how we loved each other and rejoiced with us. We accepted we had imperfections, but we worked through the issues that caused friction. It was so good doing life with someone else, someone who put me first, someone who I could feel safe with, secure and loved despite my inadequacies and failings. We were on a life journey together and I didn't feel alone, even when he was working away from home or the times I travelled with a friend to Australia. I felt so supported and validated as a person and my self-esteem grew.

We each had a house. Many people advised us to sell both and start afresh in a new house. Adrian was very clear, however, as we were sitting in my house. He said, "God wants this house."

Many years before, I felt God had asked me to give him my house. I thought I had given him everything, but I had to be very specific about giving him my house. It led to the house being used. At various times my son's friends lived with us. There wasn't a lot of room but as my daughter had married and moved out, we had a spare room. We also had church groups meeting there. On one occasion when the lounge was crowded, someone laughingly prayed for a conservatory. I didn't have any spare money at the time, and we continued to squeeze into the space we had. The house was often seen as a house of prayer and welcome, and many people commented on the peaceful atmosphere.

I was willing to sell the house and move where God and Adrian wanted to live, but God had other ideas. God gave us a vision of how he wanted the house, which exceeded my wildest imaginations. It didn't just include a conservatory; it was so much bigger and better and would need most of the money from the sale of Adrian's house. There was a delay in the sale and in that time, God spoke about the vision he had. He wanted a place where people could meet him. It would be a light in the community. He spoke of revival, including the revival of healing. It sounded awesome and exciting. I was planning to retire at the age of sixty-one and there was much to look forward to. Adrian was older by six years and continued to work past retirement age and we both retired on the same day.

Chapter 4

What's Happening?

I was excited about retirement, but Adrian didn't seem to be. His work had been exciting, rewarding and fulfilling. He had travelled the world, spoken at conferences, trained counsellors, even advised the government of Singapore on socially responsible gambling. He had made a difference to many individuals, and he loved the buzz of working away from home. He was not home-loving. I was frustrated as I wanted him to be as enthusiastic as me. I tried to be patient and understanding, and I tried to inspire him.

There were also other little niggles. Adrian didn't seem to be as capable as he used to be, and his memory wasn't so good. He took wrong turns in the car. There were little things that suggested there was a problem. He had previously had trouble with a new computer system at work. I was concerned but tried to brush it off; he was a counsellor, not a computer whizz.

Adrian grudgingly went to his GP who diagnosed him with a low-functioning thyroid. I was so relieved. Thyroxine medication would get him back on track.

It did make a slight difference but not a lot and I started to worry again.

The next time he went to the GP, he was told that he was depressed and was prescribed antidepressants, which he refused to take. I was still really worried. I wondered why he was depressed, why he couldn't see we had a mission and a ministry together, why he couldn't see that retirement was a good thing and that we could make our dream come true.

Then he was told he was pre-diabetic and then that he had type two diabetes. I didn't see how that was possible as he was fit and active and had no fat on him, but I thought maybe that was affecting him.

All the time, however, dementia was in the back of my mind. I had read Still Alice by Lisa Genova, a neuroscientist who wrote fiction based on her medical experience.[1] I loved her books, but I wished I had never read this one because it was putting unthinkable ideas in my head. There were too many similarities to the main character in the book who had been diagnosed with dementia.

There were days, however, when everything seemed OK, and I thought I was letting my imagination run away with me. We still had an enjoyable time and spent some of our retirement money on travelling. We were also involved in our church's compassion ministry, talking to people who came to our food bank, listening to them and helping them move on practically, emotionally and

---

1. Lisa Genova, *Still Alice* (Pocket Books, 2009).

spiritually. We trained volunteers and were even asked to go to another church to train their food bank volunteers. The training went well but I knew that Adrian wasn't the inspiring trainer that he had always been. He had always been a fantastic communicator but now there was something lacking.

It wasn't the best time in our relationship. We had always been honest with each other, but we didn't find it easy to talk about this; it was too frightening. I was getting frustrated and swung between getting angry and pushy and being loving and encouraging. He didn't seem to be trying very hard and I thought he was just giving up on making retirement work for us.

Other people started to notice that there was something wrong. I was, by this time, in denial, answering their concerns with "No, he is fine, thank you." I didn't want to voice my fears, as saying them out loud to someone else might make them real! My closest friends tried to help: they prayed, they encouraged, they came up with ideas and some even managed to join me in denial. Adrian didn't want to go near any doctors, saying they were making him more stressed. They kept telling him to eat a sugar-free diet to manage his diabetes better. Early on he had a memory test, which he said made him stressed. The GP, he said, was rushing him and stressing him out, which was when he was told he was depressed. He escaped into listening to music, something he always found helpful.

Eventually I asked to speak to a different GP, one who had helped me in the past and who I trusted. She was extremely popular, and we had to wait a few weeks even for a phone appointment. I was very emphatic, telling the receptionist that I didn't want to speak to anyone else and I would wait. By this time I was doing all the arranging. When the doctor phoned I explained that every time we went to see a GP Adrian was told to see the specialist diabetes doctor. I told her that I thought there was something else going on. She agreed and sent him for a brain scan. Adrian didn't want to go, and I started behaving like a mother and told him he had to go, with him moaning about it all the way. We then had to wait for the results. We saw the GP who started with a memory test. Adrian didn't do well but said it was because he got very anxious. Then she looked up the results of the brain scan and gave us the dreaded news that by this time I was expecting: Adrian's brain had shrunk and this was a classic example of dementia. Adrian didn't seem to be listening, but I heard and, although I wasn't surprised, I was devastated. Somehow we got home, and I rang my friend Cecilia to come round immediately. She knew what I was going to say. She was someone who had wanted us to share and be honest when we didn't want to talk about it. She just hugged me whilst I wept, and Adrian went back to playing his music.

Chapter 5

Let's Fight This

The GP told us that she was not allowed to give us an official diagnosis but she was sure this was dementia, so she would refer us to a memory clinic. I was sure too and stopped denying it. Now we had a diagnosis and I knew what we were facing. Instead of denying it, I was going to fight it with everything I had.

I found a book, The End of Alzheimer's by Dr Dale Bredesen.[2] The subtitle gave me so much hope: The First Programme to Prevent and Reverse the Cognitive Decline of Dementia. I bought it and read it from cover to cover. There were things that I could do to help my husband. It talked about different possible reasons why someone would be susceptible to dementia and how to reverse those conditions. I also believed in the power of prayer and knew that God healed through prayer. I was going to fight this!

I remember when Adrian and I spoke to our senior pastor, Mark. He prayed that Adrian would have a

---

2. Dr Dale Bredesen, *The End of Alzheimer's: The First Programme to Prevent and Reverse the Cognitive Decline of Dementia* (Penguin, 2017).

testimony through this. "Yes, that's it, God. Adrian will be healed of dementia and then the world will hear about it, and it will be such a witness." And I believed it would be soon. Two people independently had shared a verse with us a year earlier. "See! The winter is past; the rains are over and gone. Flowers appear on the earth; the season of singing has come" (Song of Songs 2:11-12). I thought it would mean in a few months Adrian would be healed and the doctors would be amazed. Instead, we had a long journey ahead of us.

In Dr Dale's book, I discovered several things that could have contributed to the dementia. In Adrian's university days he got into drugs, mainly LSD. He and his friends enjoyed the mind-altering experiences and thought it was fun. Adrian, though, started to become really scared of what was happening to him and phoned a Christian friend who he knew from a church youth club. "Find a quiet place and ask God to help you," advised the friend. Adrian did just that. He climbed a hill, stood there and almost yelled, "God, help me. God, help me. God, help me." God came to him and showed him he was real, and he never took drugs again. It was the beginning of Adrian's Christian walk with God. He often would share this conversion experience with others but now we wondered if the drugs were coming back to bite him. There was nothing to do about it other than to pray, which gave him a real sense of release. I hoped this was a start of the healing process. Adrian too was enthusiastic and wanted to use this experience to give talks to young people and warn them of the dangers of drugs.

I read many books, especially by people who believed that dementia could be reversed or at least halted. We stopped eating sugar and gluten, cooked in coconut oil, ate good fats and organic fruit and vegetables, bought supplements and liberally added herbs and spices. One book said that medicinal cannabis could help, another said that inflammation was a factor, and that tooth decay could cause problems, so we ate anti-inflammatory foods and visited the dentist. We bought probiotics and grew our own kefir, which I made into milkshakes using coconut milk.

I was so encouraged when we went to the memory clinic to talk to the consultant. As we waited, I spotted Dr Dale Bredesen's book on the bookshelf of her office. She had the book – The End of Alzheimer's. I told her that we had bought the book and were following as much of it as we were able without going to the USA to see Dr Dale. The consultant was encouraging but cautious. She felt that the diet was a healthy one and that it wouldn't do any harm, and that the supplements were OK but warned us about spending loads of money on some of the other practices, which I had already dismissed. She advised us to spend our money on a holiday together and enjoy ourselves. Other people, too, thought we should just make the most of the time. "Walk in the park and buy an ice cream," was one person's advice. Yes, we walked but no, I wasn't going to put sugar into Adrian's body. I was going to beat this!

There was medication Adrian could take that didn't cure the dementia but could halt some of the symptoms.

I wished we knew about this before and would have asked for it earlier. Again, though, this seemed like something positive.

I used my teaching skills. As a special needs teacher, I decided that I could teach Adrian some of the skills he had forgotten, breaking down the skills into small steps, encouraging him to relearn. I was going to do everything in my power for my husband and I was not going to be passive! I was on a mission, and nothing was going to beat me!

Most of all I believed that God could do the impossible. I believed with my whole heart that he would heal Adrian. He protected my daughter in the womb, he could heal my husband. Many people joined us in prayer, and we waited for the miracle that would happen.

One of my friends, Jo, was concerned about the amount of pressure I was putting on us both. One of the causes of dementia suggested by my research was constant stress, something that Adrian was prone to. He loved living on adrenaline and my manic attempt at bringing healing was probably not doing either of us any good. We still ate healthily and continued the supplements, but I relaxed a bit, prayed and tried to live as normally as possible. It wasn't easy but the relief of letting go helped us both.

We decided to take the advice of the consultant. Adrian and I loved travelling. We had plans to go to India, but Adrian couldn't face that, so we went on a cruise to the Caribbean, a trip we had done before. We knew we would have easy transfers from the plane to the ship and we knew what to expect, so we booked it. We set sail in January 2020. I had to do the arrangements, carry the tickets and passports and ensure we were in the right place at the right time. Adrian was willing to carry a card with him saying that he had dementia, and which cabin we were in if he needed help. I was so proud of him for acknowledging this. We had a good holiday, and we overcame any difficulties. Adrian loved dancing and he was in his element dancing to the sounds of the Caribbean. He had so much energy and flexibility and many people applauded his moves. Again, I was so proud of him and so pleased he was enjoying himself.

Adrian had always been attentive to my needs, and I was grateful that he still was. I wanted to go swimming in the sea, and he sat on the beach watching as he wasn't keen on swimming. I was also incredibly grateful to a couple who realised his dementia and supported me a few times when I needed it. On one occasion whilst I was swimming Adrian felt a few drops of rain and decided to move. The couple ensured he was safe as I quickly got out of the water. People were exceedingly kind and understanding and we had a good holiday despite the responsibility I felt at times.

At this time, we were in a rented flat whilst our house was being renovated. Adrian, despite his dementia, was happy with this and understood why we were there. I decided that in a few months' time, by June, when we were due to be back in our house, Adrian would be healed and we would start a new ministry to the community around us. Every night as we cuddled up in bed, I would place my hands on Adrian's head and pray with such faith against the tau tangles, amyloid plaques and other symptoms of dementia, and ask the Holy Spirit to come and bring life back to the neural pathways and brain cells.

Adrian was coping with the dementia and was happy going out for walks, to the shops, helping at our church food bank and Care Centre, seeing friends and family and going to church. He had always loved dancing and music, but his interest peeked. Our church had a vibrant worship band and Adrian lost all inhibitions as he danced in worship at the front. We also went to regular concerts, which he thoroughly enjoyed, although I had to stop him from getting up and dancing on the stage.

I still had faith; faith that God would heal Adrian and that we would have a powerful ministry together. This time would pass and when we got back to our renovated house all would be well.

Chapter 6

Then Covid Hit Us

Covid hit all of us hard, but Adrian found it particularly difficult.

"Are we going to Vineyard today?" Adrian asked. Vineyard was the name of our church.

"No, we are not allowed," I replied. I tried to explain about the coronavirus and that we were only allowed out for walks and shopping.

"Are we seeing the family?"

I tried to explain again.

"Where are we going then?"

"Who are we seeing?"

It was so difficult to explain something that we all were grappling with. Adrian had always loved being with people. When we went to the supermarket we had to queue and to keep two metres away from people. He found it difficult and was confused and I felt like a nagging wife.

Explaining that it was not safe to be with people because of the virus caused Adrian more problems. He picked up on the "not safe" and started believing that everywhere was unsafe. He thought the cars were unsafe and that we shouldn't be going out. He started to get really anxious. I insisted that everywhere was safe and tried to reassure him, but then he wanted to go near people again. It was so hard.

I have heard many stories of people becoming mentally unwell in the Covid years. I saw it first hand when Adrian started talking to his friend in the mirror. He insisted it wasn't himself and that it was his friend, despite me showing him both of us in the mirror. Whenever I said we were going out Adrian would ask his friend if he was coming. Sometimes I left him to it as the day was long and there wasn't much else for him to do, and he seemed really happy and not disturbed by it. Then it escalated and Adrian started seeing or hearing less-friendly people. It came to a head when he thought someone was threatening to kill him.

I was so grateful for the support we had at that time. We had a caring GP who phoned back immediately when I called. She had informed the receptionist to let her know whenever I phoned and needed help. I also had a close friend, Cecilia, who I could call at any time.

One Saturday morning Adrian started shouting – "Don't kill me! Stop, don't kill me!" It was awful seeing him so scared and distressed. At the time we were on the second floor of a small block of flats. Due to Covid no one could come and visit. I phoned Cecilia who came running. She stood in the road outside with me looking through the open window at the same time as I was on the phone to the GP. Cecilia prayed and supported me until Adrian calmed down and the imaginary person had disappeared. The GP prescribed olanzapine. She also gave us lorazepam to use until the olanzapine kicked in. The medication made a difference and Adrian became a lot calmer.

Some of the time I was coping surprisingly well. I was optimistic about Adrian being healed and I still had faith in God's ability to do the impossible. I was also holding on to the fact that we would soon be moving back to our renovated house and that Covid would not last forever.

At other times, I felt so stressed. I felt ashamed of the times when I was impatient with Adrian. I tried to be calm and understanding but I didn't always manage it as it was hard to be cooped up in a flat together. I had to help Adrian wash, which wasn't easy as he often resisted getting in the bath or shower and he hated having his hair washed. He needed help in the night to go to the toilet, which I didn't mind but I found it extremely difficult if he just aimlessly wandered about whilst I was trying to sleep. He often resisted getting dressed or into bed and sometimes he refused to eat and started losing weight. One night I was so stressed I shouted at him and then hit him. I didn't hurt him, but he was so shocked. I nearly didn't confess to this, but I am a human being, and I didn't plan to do it. I was so frustrated, and I thought he was deliberately making it difficult for me, which of course he wasn't. I was shocked, too, as well as feeling really guilty. It was many months later that I forgave myself.

One of the things that kept me going was how well the house renovations were going. Many projects were delayed due to the difficulty with staff sickness, lack of materials and other Covid-related issues. One of the electricians working on our house was amazed at the progress of our house. He said, "I'm not a religious man but someone up there is looking after this project. It is the only one in the area that hasn't had delays." He wasn't surprised when I told him that it was a very prayed-over house and that we wanted God to use it as a place of refuge and healing.

Clark, our project manager, was really enthusiastic and such a perfectionist. He put his heart and soul into the job, as well as his incredible skills and creative thinking. I insisted that Adrian accompanied me on daily walks to get us out of the flat. We arranged with Cecilia to stop at her house, where she looked out of her open window whilst we stood on the other side of her hedge and talked and prayed. Then we walked on to our house, where we could watch the transformation taking place.

The day came when, from the outside, the house looked complete. Clark said he was not allowing me inside until the interior was finished and decorated, as he wanted to give me the "wow!" factor when I walked in. He wanted me to enjoy it first without Adrian, as by this time Adrian was confused, didn't like standing still and needed my constant attention. Cecilia, my daughter Lisa, and one of our pastors, Trevor, took Adrian to Cecilia's house while I was given the keys to our "new" house. It was awesome and I walked around it open-mouthed.

Later I was joined by the others, and I asked Trevor to pray for the house and for complete healing for Adrian. I was excited and hopeful.

Moving into our "new" house was such a joy. I had decided that I wasn't going to just stuff our belongings into cupboards but was going to take my time to throw out anything we didn't need. We also had some new tables and chairs that needed to be put together; we needed to think about pictures for the walls and where to put our furniture and other belongings. Whilst we were in the flat I had little to do so I could spend time with Adrian; now I wanted to use my time to make our house a home, but Adrian didn't really understand the need and I became very frustrated. He loved the house, though, and said on one occasion, "I love it here. I could live here." I reassured him that this was our home and that we did live here. At first, I thought this was going to be the start of Adrian being more settled as we had more space than in the flat, as well as a garden and all our belongings, including his vinyls and record player.

Adrian felt safe in the house and was content, but he didn't want to go out as he thought it was unsafe outside, even in the garden. At this time, the Covid rules were that we could have friends in the garden but not inside the house. I was so pleased to see friends and family in the garden, but Adrian was distressed and tried to persuade us to go inside as he was genuinely concerned for our safety. Then he started talking to the mirror again, seemingly seeing or hearing his imaginative friend.

One of my friends, Anne, was supportive. She asked me whether Adrian was taking a certain medication for dementia. I responded that he was, and she suggested I look at the possible side effects. She explained that her father had been on the medication and that he started hallucinating, but once he stopped the medication the hallucinations disappeared. Sure enough, hallucinations were a possible side effect, so I phoned the doctor who said that this medication did not suit everybody and, in fact, as the dementia had advanced it probably was not helping anyway. I was again hopeful as we stopped the medication but unfortunately it didn't make any difference.

I loved my house but staying in didn't suit me and I was getting more and more frustrated as I wanted to go out. I also wanted to buy things for the house, and I wanted to make the house a home. This wasn't what I had planned. I had genuinely believed that when we moved back in Adrian would be better, but now he wouldn't go out and I couldn't leave him. I cried out for help. My brother came to stay for a few days; was a much-needed emotional support and helped me sort out the house. Friends from our church came and almost pushed me out of the door so I could get time away from the house and Adrian. I felt so blessed to have had that support as I was just trying to survive each day. I cried out to God, questioning him why Adrian was getting worse, not better.

The time came when I had to face that I was not coping. My next-door neighbour, a community mental health nurse for the elderly, who had been so helpful throughout, came round one evening looking concerned. She gave me a kind but firm lecture on burn out and said I needed help. It was a wake-up call – one I didn't like. She gave me some numbers to call, which were helpful but there were restrictions on what help was available because of Covid. In the end a psychiatrist came round to see us. Trevor asked to attend as well. Despite being a gentle and quiet man, he stated very forcibly that, as my church pastor, he was responsible for my health and well-being and that I needed help. I was touched by his care and felt so blessed to be part of the church family. Respite care was suggested, and I phoned the appropriate number and spoke to a kind and considerate lady. She said that we would have to pay for any respite care and advised me to look for a place and contact homes personally as it would be much quicker than relying on them. I knew I couldn't cope but I also dreaded the thought of putting my husband, my soulmate, the one I had promised lasting devotion to, in a care home. I reassured myself that it would temporary. Although I was a very capable and organised person, at this point I was so overwhelmed, tired and confused that I couldn't face the task of looking for care homes. In fact, I didn't need to as my son Geoff, with my friends Anne and Sandra organised me, looked up websites and told me what phone numbers to write down.

We didn't get as far as respite, however, despite finding a suitable place, as Adrian stopped washing and shaving and was becoming more distressed. There was no way he would go near water, and I could not persuade or force him. It all came to a head when Adrian started shouting and trying to defend himself from an imaginary attacker who was trying to kill him. My friend Anne took control and phoned 111. On hearing what was happening the telephonist said she was calling the police. It all seemed to be taken out of my hands.

The police were kind, gentle and respectful. They appeared relaxed but I could see they were also being vigilant, observing Adrian discretely. They were really sorry that this was the only way to get help at the moment due to Covid. Then the paramedics arrived, who were equally supportive. After sitting with us for quite a while they said they needed to take Adrian to hospital. Due to Covid restrictions I should not have been allowed to go but because of Adrian's distress they allowed me to go and to stay with him in the A&E department.

I will always remember the love that Adrian showed to me on that day. The only way we could get Adrian out of the house and into the ambulance was to tell him that I needed to go to hospital and ask him if he would go with me. He overcame his fears for my benefit and willingly got into the ambulance with me, despite mumbling that we were all going to die. I knew he loved me but that was extraordinary!

It's all such a blur looking back. I think I just went through the motions, doing what I needed to do to support Adrian and get him the help he needed. I couldn't even worry about how distressed he was at the hospital. I couldn't cope anymore and needed someone to take over. We needed professional help.

Chapter 7

Relief and Distress

I felt relief when Adrian was sectioned and kept in hospital. I couldn't even feel guilty or worried about him being distressed, I just had to let him go.

My daughter Lisa was brilliant. She was with me when Adrian and I were taken to the hospital, then stayed behind, cleaned up and sorted out food for when I got home. It took a few hours before I could leave, and Adrian was taken from A&E and found a room, where he was given support and a bed before being transferred to an elderly mental health unit. Lisa picked me up from the hospital, fed me, listened to me, and took me for a walk when I became agitated. I was tired but restless as I probably had adrenalin pumping around my body.

Due to Covid, Adrian had to stay for two weeks in a unit that had been temporarily named as an admission unit to ensure he didn't have the virus. During that time I wasn't allowed to see him. I had such mixed feelings. I was so exhausted that I was glad that someone else was looking after him. It was a relief, but I also wanted to show him that I hadn't abandoned him and let him down. I wanted to make sure he was alright. In a way it was good that I didn't have a choice.

The next few days went past in a blur, but six days after Adrian had initially been taken to A&E I got a phone call. By this time he had been in the unit for a few days. It was the consultant who started the conversation by asking if I had family with me. "No," I replied, "but I do have a close friend here." I was alarmed as he started talking.

"Expect the worst," he told me. "Adrian is not eating or drinking, and we are not allowed to force him."

"What do you mean?" I asked. "Do you mean he will die?"

"He has advanced dementia so I am sure he wouldn't want to live," replied the consultant.

I was flabbergasted and questioned how long. "It could be days or hours." I was in shock but managed to ask if I should come, but he said that I could not because of Covid until it was an emergency. It sounded like one to me but there was nothing I could do.

I phoned Lisa but there was no answer, so I phoned her husband, Neil. "She's at the hairdresser but I will get her straightaway," he answered. "She will be with you a.s.a.p."

I imagined him running into the hairdresser and grabbing my daughter halfway through her haircut so I told him to wait until she came home, which would probably be in twenty minutes. I knew that they had plans for the weekend, but he said they could be cancelled and reassured me that she definitely would come. After supporting me the weekend before, working full time in the week and looking after her two boys, she would be willing to drive one and a half hours to be with me. I was so grateful.

That night, not surprisingly, I couldn't sleep so I spent most of it praying for Adrian. It was the only thing I could do. I had asked others to pray too.

At 6am I was desperate to know how Adrian was, so I decided to phone the unit as I knew they would have night staff on duty. I explained to the nurse who answered the phone what the consultant had said. "I'm sure he didn't say that," she replied. She looked up in the notes and there it was, in black and white. "He did," she said and read out what he had written, "and there is a 'do not resuscitate' order." She said that she was shocked as she was sitting eating toast and drinking tea with Adrian before he went to bed. "He didn't seem like he was dying," she stated. I was so relieved but explained that I had not agreed to a DNR. Evidently I must have done, although in my shock I had no idea what I might have agreed to. I needed more information before I would agree to a DNR, and she agreed to ask the consultant to phone me on Monday.

Lisa heard me talking and came downstairs. After a while I went back to bed and this time I slept. Lisa was attentive and kept looking in on me to make sure I was alright. Our roles had reversed, and I experienced her as the good mum she was to her two sons.

The road through dementia was feeling like a nightmare and such an up-and-down experience. Over the years I felt that I was on a roller coaster of emotions and experiences. I never knew how Adrian would be and what to expect next. This was still only the beginning of the journey we were to take through this awful disease!

Chapter 8

Professional Help

I was convinced that the combination of dementia and Covid had caused Adrian's psychotic symptoms. As well as being relieved that someone else was looking after Adrian, I also wanted him to have the expertise of someone with experience of mental health. There had been a lot of media coverage about the increase of mental health issues throughout Covid and I was convinced this wasn't just dementia that we were dealing with.

After Adrian's two-week stay in the assessment unit, he was moved to a different unit that was on the other side of the county. I was so concerned about him having to get into the hospital transport as I thought he would be frightened and confused. As I was not allowed to be with him, I prayed most of the day. The staff at the first unit had encouraged me with stories of Adrian dancing, eating and drinking. He had started medication that was helping and there was a lovely registrar who talked me through what was happening. I felt supported and I knew Adrian was too. Now he had to start again with different staff in a different environment. I needn't have worried, though, as the staff had experience and skills and knew what they were doing, ensuring that Adrian had a successful transition and settled into the new unit.

After a few days I was told I could visit Adrian, but due to Covid it had to be in the garden. I was looking forward to seeing him, but I was worried about the visit, whether he wanted to see me and whether he would be distressed in the garden. The staff gave him some medication to calm him a little but not enough to sedate him, and it was such a beautiful visit. We spent two hours on a bench in the garden together, talking and holding hands. One of the things he said to me was that everything he had was mine. We also prayed together, awesome and real prayers. This was the start of many vastly different visits, some good, others awful. Many times, Adrian would not go into the garden. On some occasions he was taken into the garden by staff, but he kept knocking on the door to be let back in. He tried to take me inside, but I had to tell him I was not allowed. On some occasions he told me not to be silly, he would take me in. Sometimes I stood at the open French doors and looked in where he would be sitting two metres away in line with Covid regulations. Sometimes he just got up and walked off. He often asked the staff where I was but then ignored me. I had to understand and accept that this was not him but the dementia, but it was difficult.

There were also challenging times when the consultant was trying different combinations of medications. He was a hardworking, committed man who was determined to get the best possible outcome for his patients. He told me he could not cure dementia, but he wanted to give his patients a good quality of life, so he wanted to find the best medication for Adrian. He told me that Adrian would not be coming home and that he needed dementia nursing care. He wanted the best place for Adrian, and he warned me this might not be the nearest to me. He also wanted somewhere where Adrian could stay long term, so he didn't have to have any more changes. I knew Adrian was in good hands. I knew there was no way we could manage at home, and I trusted this man to do the best for my husband.

Adrian always loved being with people and one of the real difficulties with being at home during Covid was the lack of contact with other people. On some occasions when I was looking through the doors of the unit, I could see Adrian interacting with other residents around the table. He was not unhappy.

Adrian and I had dreaded the idea of him going into a care home. We had agreed we would do everything possible to prevent it and cope at home but now I knew this was the right move. It helped that I didn't get a choice as Adrian was legally detained and it was not up to me what happened to him. The consultant said that I wasn't to choose the home for Adrian as I wouldn't know what to look for. He wanted the best and most appropriate place for his patients, which might not be the nearest and most convenient for me. Not wanting to be passive, however, I researched what was available even if I didn't get to choose. The consultant mentioned one possible place, so I looked into it.

My next-door neighbour, the mental health nurse for the elderly, recommended I look at a particular home. She said that a lot of her patients seemed to do well there, and it had an outstanding review by the Care Quality Commission (CQC). Unfortunately, due to Covid, most places were not accepting visitors, so a lot of my research was done online, and I emailed a few homes. This particular one was the only one that invited me for a chat, even though I could not walk around inside. I was really impressed. The thing that struck me most was that there was a consistency of staff. The manager boasted that she had never lost staff in the ten years she had been working there, except for personal reasons. No one seemed to move on because they were unhappy, and they very rarely had to advertise for staff and never had to resort to using agency staff. To me, that spoke volumes.

The consultant invited me to a meeting to discuss the next steps with a group of professionals who had worked with Adrian. Evidently, they had had many people move successfully to this particular home and the consultant said it would meet Adrian's needs and was very willing for him to go there as it was similar to the one he had initially mentioned. It was also much easier for me to visit, which I know was not the consideration but was a bonus. There would be an assessment by the home and funding would have to be approved. I was so impressed with the way it all happened and how all the professionals worked together. I was allocated a social worker who was really helpful, and it was all sorted in a couple of weeks. Adrian was granted continuing health care paid for by the NHS but as I had chosen a home that was more expensive than the basic home, I was required to fund the extra cost, which I was able and willing to do. I was so grateful for the way all the professionals involved were so committed to getting it right for Adrian. I believe God was in it too. Later I spoke to a lady who lived down our street. "It is so hard getting the right care home, isn't it, and so many hurdles to overcome. It is such a nightmare." My experience was the opposite, so I am very thankful.

Covid was still with us. There were restrictions throughout the country but even more so in care homes. Initially I couldn't see Adrian at all but then I was allowed to see him through a window in a tiny room in the reception area. Faye, a lovely, caring, activity leader brought him down in the lift, ensured he had plenty of tea and biscuits and sat with him during our visit, but he was so confused and didn't like being shut in the room. He also didn't like the lift and I am not sure he even was aware of me most of the time. Faye was very reassuring and held his hand and, on some occasions, Adrian calmed and placed his hands on the window in order to connect with me. I was so pleased with that connection, but it was so, so painful being separated by glass, so close but so far away. It was surreal, so hard and yet so wonderful when I felt he recognised me and on occasions spoke to me through the microphone. I have no idea what he knew or what he felt. I knew, though, that the visits were sometimes frightening to him, and he wanted to go back upstairs to familiarity. Faye encouraged him to stay but then terminated the visit if he was distressed.

On one occasion, after Faye took Adrian upstairs, she ran after me and found me sitting in my car where I was feeling distressed and upset, trying to get myself together enough to drive. She was so kind and understanding and thought of a way our visits could be better. Adrian was on the first floor but as the home was on a slope his room, which was round the back, looked out to ground level. Along the corridor was the pub, which evidently Adrian liked. She suggested I could walk round the back across the grass and look through the pub window at the back, which would be a lot better for Adrian who was happy sitting in a comfortable chair with a pot of tea and some biscuits. He found it difficult, however, to relate to me through the window and many times I just chatted with Faye who sat stroking Adrian's hands. I think he enjoyed the visits even though I didn't know if he even remembered me most of the time. It was heart-breaking. Faye said she felt guilty that she could touch Adrian and give him hugs when I couldn't, but I reassured her that I was pleased that she was giving comfort to him. Sometimes Adrian would not stay in the pub and wandered out into the corridor. On one occasion the visit had to be through the window of his room. On this occasion Adrian was frustrated with the carer who brought him. "What am I doing in here?" he demanded. He didn't like sitting in his room and associated it with going to bed so he left me standing grieving outside.

Adrian loved his tea and biscuits. He also liked puddings and porridge, but he would not eat dinners. Then one day he stopped wanting anything. I was warned that this might be him moving to the next stage of dementia and I should be prepared for the worst. The brain might now have forgotten how to recognise hunger and how to eat food. Instead of feeling downhearted I went into battle mode, asking God to heal him. I think staff probably saw it as denial and that I was not accepting the severity of the situation, but I saw the red kites overhead and I felt that God was carrying me on eagles' wings, as it says in the Bible. In fact, Adrian had an infection and after a day or two of antibiotics started eating and drinking better.

Adrian's birthday was in December, a few days after Christmas. I was standing outside the pub window with snow falling on me. I had brought a present and a card a few days earlier so they could be kept in quarantine for 72 hours. Faye brought in a cake, my present and card and we sang "Happy Birthday" to him. Adrian smiled and I was so pleased that he had responded to our celebrating, but I was also so sad as I remembered previous birthday trips to London, dinner in the Hard Rock Café followed by a trip to the theatre.

I think that as everyone was struggling because of Covid, my situation sometimes didn't seem so bad. I was in a support bubble with my son Geoff and his family, and I was able to enjoy my two young granddaughters. Adrian was safe and didn't have to worry about Covid in the same way as the rest of the world. I decided that

God was protecting Adrian and that when Covid was over, he would heal him.

As we all had to cope with Covid there was a type of camaraderie that connected us all, which prevented me from feeling totally isolated. I, like many others, used a variety of coping strategies, some good, some not so good and maybe some unhealthy, but I got through the Covid months. As other people were facing difficulties, I sometimes didn't feel my situation was so different from those of the general population. It was difficult for all of us, and I proceeded to find ways to manage each day.

I kept myself busy, knitting doll's clothes for my granddaughters, helping them with home schooling, taking a disabled friend's dog out for a walk each day, and continuing to write blogs and a training pack for young people with special needs. I was even asked to record a training video, which kept me busy.

I also felt the pull to numb feelings, which I did by playing computer games and drinking more alcohol than usual. Not healthy but I did it.

One of the positives during this time was that we all discovered Zoom and WhatsApp. I was thrilled to have so many friends who I could talk to and many of my relationships became more intimate and real despite not being able to meet in person.

Many people advised me to join a dementia support group. I knew they could be really helpful, but I could not face listening to other people's stories. Maybe it would make Adrian's dementia seem too real and I did not want to think about possible future difficulties. I was blessed to have so many friends and family who were supportive and often phoned me. Talking helped me such a lot and I would encourage anyone facing the dementia of a loved one to get as much support as possible and try not to be self-sufficient.

The Coronavirus pandemic started to wane, and life was becoming more normal for most people. There was now limited visiting within the care home, and I was able to book an appointment to see Adrian inside the home for half an hour every two weeks. This time between visits seemed so spaced out and the time short. We had to check in, do a Covid test, put on PPE and have our temperatures taken. Then we had to be escorted to a room, usually the resident's bedroom, although I was allowed to use the pub as Adrian was more comfortable there. The limited time was bad enough, but it was devastating when after looking forward to it, Adrian walked off, was sleepy or needed the toilet. Sometimes I just wanted to scream.

Gradually the visits became more frequent and longer.

Then the Omicron variant appeared, and restrictions were increased again.

I can only describe this period as a roller coaster. Visits were planned, then cancelled. Visits happened but left me in despair when Adrian didn't seem to even recognise me. Visits were brilliant and Adrian was pleased to see me and told me I was beautiful and he loved me. Visits were frustrating because Adrian would not sit down and wanted to walk in the corridor, where I wasn't allowed to go in order to protect other residents from possible infection. There were also times when staff or residents tested positive for Covid, and no visits were allowed. In early 2022 many people tested positive for Covid often without symptoms. Each time the home was closed, and I thought I would never be able to see Adrian. I yelled to God in frustration. Then I received a phone call asking me if I would be Adrian's essential carer as the manager of the home thought that Adrian was missing me and would appreciate it if I came in three times a week to help him with his meals. I jumped at the idea and readily agreed to have a weekly PCR test, get some training, book the times I was coming and stay in his room away from other residents. Fortunately, Adrian was happier in his room and was willing to eat his meals there.

Sometimes these times were encouraging as our relationship was still there and there was a connection between us. It was as though our love bypassed the brain but was felt on a heart-to-heart or soul-to-soul basis. I knew that Adrian knew me and loved me, even though I didn't think he even knew my name. He rarely said anything and when I spoke, I didn't know if he understood, but he sensed my love. I gave him head and shoulder massages, held his hands and prayed. He seemed to feel peace and I am sure that he had experienced God's love.

Adrian had stopped feeding himself unless it was to hold a biscuit or a cup of tea, so I needed to feed him with a spoon. I was happy to do that, especially when he seemed to enjoy the food. I was just pleased to be there. Then it suddenly hit me: I was feeding my husband like a baby! It was even worse, though, when he wouldn't eat and pushed me away. I vehemently questioned God, wanting to know what he was doing and why Adrian was getting worse and not better.

Then Adrian got Covid, and I was not able to see him. I phoned up regularly to see how he was and was usually told that he was poorly and in bed, that he was weak and frail but not in immediate danger. The staff were great but many of them were sick too, and those who were well were struggling to isolate and care for the many sick residents. I trusted the staff, but I was really worried that Adrian would feel isolated and not understand why he could not leave his room. Then I got Covid, and the time of separation extended even further. By the time I was clear to visit I had no idea what I was expecting. I was afraid that Adrian would not recognise me, that he was distressed or that Covid had caused a further deterioration in his physical and mental health.

Adrian in fact looked well, was pleased to see me and seemed settled. I was relieved and I continued the essential-care role. I was grateful but underneath I was seething. I didn't want to be his carer; I wanted to be his soulmate, his lover and his wife.

Chapter 9

Help is Available

I had always suffered from digestive problems and IBS (irritable bowel syndrome) but had learned to control it through diet and occasional medication. Now, though, it was getting worse, and I was also getting pains under my ribs and acid reflux or heartburn. I began to think maybe I had something serious.

Just as I was beginning to get anxious, there was a word of knowledge at church. A team of people pray before the service and God gives them words or pictures about ailments he wants to heal. On this occasion someone said that God wanted to touch someone who had ongoing digestive problems. I responded and was prayed for by a lovely lady called Anny, who seemed to hear from God. She didn't pray much about digestion but said that my soul was weary. She prayed about the weariness and also gave me a lot of encouragement about how special I was to God, how valued I was and about future hope in my life. I realised I had been bottling up a lot of feelings. I had tried to get on with life, but all the unfelt feelings were building up in my stomach and yes, I was weary inside.

I later asked to meet up with Anny, who was a spiritual director, a title she did not like as she said she didn't direct anyone but just walked beside people on their spiritual journeys. I had to wait to see her as she was going abroad to visit her family, but I was looking forward to talking with her as I thought she might be able to help. Anny did help, not in the way I had imagined though. She suggested that I didn't need spiritual direction but help with my grief. I needed emotional help, not spiritual help. This made loads of sense to me. Anny was a retired psychotherapist and said that if she was working with me as a therapist, she would want to address the grief. She suggested I see a counsellor or therapist. I had had therapy in the past when I had learned to identify and manage my feelings, but I realised that the feelings I had now were different and more complex. I had not thought of seeing a therapist, but I knew this was the answer to my next steps. I looked online and a therapist jumped off the page. He responded to my email immediately and had one slot available, which I readily accepted.

Sometimes there were signs that Adrian was getting better. Carers greeted me with good news on a regular basis:

"He was talking!"

"He answered a question!"

"He used the toilet!"

"He was smiling and laughing!"

"He joined in an activity!"

Then the most exciting, a carer greeted me with "You must watch this!" She showed me a video of Adrian dancing with her. Adrian loved dancing in the past but had not danced for the last eighteen months or so. This video demonstrated that he had not forgotten the moves he used to make that always brought applause from anyone watching.

I was thrilled and went to find Adrian. He was not in the least interested in seeing me and in fact didn't seem to recognise me. I was so disappointed after hearing the good news, that the connection between us didn't seem to be there. The next two visits were equally as bad and yet there was so much excitement coming from the staff team. I knew I should be excited and pleased, but I felt abandoned, lost, confused, sad, angry and jealous. I felt like giving up, but I knew I wouldn't. I wanted Adrian to be happy and settled so I was pleased that he was relating to the staff, and he seemed at home and comfortable, but I was grieving. Whenever he seemed to connect, I was ecstatic; when he said that I was beautiful or lovely or that he loved me, it made my day, and I started craving that whenever I visited. Covid restrictions had been lifted and most people were getting on with their lives, but my life seemed mundane and routine, full of sorrow and despair.

My friend Jo woke in the middle of the night with a message she thought was from God: "Bless what I am doing." I was trying to control, to pray harder, to encourage Adrian to recognise me, to push Adrian to remember, to prove to the carers that I also could see the improvement in my husband. They in turn were encouraging Adrian to talk to me and to dance and to smile. Adrian had never responded to pressure like that, even in the past when he was healthy. I let go and instead of pleading with God, I just said, "God, I bless what you are doing in Adrian's life." It was in fact a relief and a release as I stopped striving and struggling. The next day I visited, Adrian was sitting in his room. He saw me and smiled a really warm smile of welcome, pleasure and recognition. "You look amazing," I told him. "Have you had your hair cut?" He nodded and looked really proud of himself. The next two hours were incredible. Adrian talked a lot, often single words or phrases but all addressed to me. He told me how much he liked me and what a wonderful person I was and how lovely I was. We even managed a few kisses. While I was feeding him, I gazed into the distance. "Are you OK?" he asked. He had always picked up on my feelings and moods in the past. This was wonderful; not only did he recognise me, he was caring for me!

The problem with dementia, though, is that each day is different. Sometimes I just couldn't wait to leave as it was so difficult, and other times I held on to the positives.

Adrian loved having his head and shoulders massaged. It was so good to feel I was doing something for him that he liked. It was so good when he said "lovely" when I massaged him. It was so encouraging when he enjoyed his food, and I could report to the staff that he had eaten it all. It pleased me when he enjoyed his cup of tea. It was brilliant when there seemed to be some conversation, even in single words. It was wonderful if he said he loved me. I craved it but it didn't happen all the time. I had rejoiced in any improvement or isolated good day, even rejoicing in him opening his bowels in the toilet instead of in his pad. I was pleased that I could visit whenever I wanted and for as long as I wanted, and I started to visit most days. Covid was essentially over. I had longed to be able to see Adrian more often and had yearned and prayed for the positives I was seeing. The positives were now not enough, though, and suddenly I realised I was facing an ongoing situation. I had coped in the crisis but now the "ongoingness" (an expression that I think should be in the dictionary) was facing me. This was my husband we were talking about. We were rejoicing that my husband who had spoken at international conferences was doing a poo in the toilet! I wanted to scream!

This was where my therapy started! My feelings were starting to be unbottled and expressed. It was both freeing and frightening.

Grief

The grief cycle is usually associated with death, the death of a loved one. With dementia, there is a profound sense of loss but the person being grieved is not dead. Sometimes I thought it would be easier to cope with the grief if he was dead, but I didn't want that. Some people say that you have lost the person even if they are still alive. My experience was that there was still something of that person. He was not just a brain; he was a whole person who related emotionally with his heart. I didn't always see it, but I did experience who he used to be and still was on occasions. That gave me hope and joy despite the intense sadness I also felt.

My therapy often addressed this dichotomy. I was grieving but my husband was still alive. Colin, my therapist, talked about it as the limbo of grief. I had started grieving when I first recognised the symptoms of dementia, but I was also fighting against the grief. In some ways I was in limbo, with no sense of resolution. Instead, I was on a roller coaster of despair, hope, love and even joy. There was no ending, just a continuous "up and downness" – another expression I think should be in the dictionary!

Although each stage of the grief cycle may appear at various times there is a sense of going through the stages until there is some kind of resolution. But with dementia there are so many nuances and complications in the process.

The five stages of grief, suggested by psychiatrist Elisabeth Kübler-Ross, are:

1. Denial

2. Anger

3. Bargaining

4. Depression

5. Acceptance

The first stage of grief is usually denial. I am not sure if I was in denial when I saw progress, when there were some signs that Adrian was getting better, when I believed that God was answering my prayers and those of many others. He was possibly just more settled and no longer experienced the mental distress that accompanied the Covid pandemic with all the uncertainty and fear. I certainly was in denial at the beginning of this journey when I didn't want to see or name the symptoms, but by this time I did know that Adrian had advanced dementia. He was not dead, though, and therefore where there was life there was hope and, ultimately, complete healing. Many people said that I needed to come to terms with Adrian's dementia. They probably thought I was in denial, but I was not. I knew he had dementia. I saw it when I fed him with a spoon, when I changed him when he had done a poo in his pads, when he didn't respond to me, when he shuffled seemingly aimlessly around the corridor. I heard it when I read the Deprivation of Liberty assessment or the social worker's annual report. I felt it when he didn't seem to know who I was and never used my name. I knew it when I couldn't share my life with him and I couldn't explain my life to him; when the only life I had with him was in a nursing home and I left the rest of my life outside the door. I knew it and I was not denying it, even though I was hoping for healing. I was believing what the Bible said, "Jesus Christ is the same yesterday and today and forever" (Hebrews 13:8). I had believed Jesus healed people in Bible times, but I had also experienced healing in the present day. I knew in my heart that God could heal so there was no reason why he could not heal Adrian.

The second stage is anger. The very fact that I believed God could heal made me so angry. I was angry that my hopes for the future that Adrian and I planned together were not happening. I was also angry with Adrian for not trying harder to get better. And I was angry with life that was so cruel. I told myself to be thankful for the care he was getting, for any small connection or achievement, for the memories of the good times we had together. I remembered and was thankful for all we had and did but I wanted more. "Memories are of dead people," I wanted to scream. "But he is not dead, he is alive, and I want more life with him."

I knew I was bottling up my feelings. Throughout my therapy I kept coming back to my stomach pains, my digestive difficulties, and each time a feeling that I had suppressed would start to emerge. All through my life I had bottled up my feelings, often not realising it, but my stomach knew. My stomach felt the unexpressed emotions that I often unconsciously buried. In my first session with Colin, my therapist, I said I wanted to cry but somehow the tears would not flow and the sobbing I craved didn't happen. I thought that if only I could cry, I would feel better. Even though Adrian was not dead I was going through grief, and I assumed that grief should involve crying, and crying would bring relief. Although I had cried on rare occasions, I think I was holding myself together to fight this cruel disease, to focus on being there for my husband, my soulmate. I wasn't going to be defeated and I was not going to give in or fall apart, not while Adrian was still alive. As I worked with Colin, an overwhelming sense of anger rose from the depths of my being. My whole body was angry. I wanted to scream, stamp my feet, thump my fists and lie on the floor having a full-blown temper tantrum. I wanted to shout and yell from the top of a mountain, yelling to the furthest ocean and beyond. I was not sad so much as furious with the cruelty of life, with dementia, with the heartache and the slow decline I was seeing. I did not know that I was so angry, but my stomach knew and was holding the anger until this time when I felt safe and able to express it.

The third stage of grief is bargaining, which often includes a sense of guilt. I consistently said that I didn't feel guilty. Many people told me not to feel guilty about Adrian going into a care home, but I didn't feel guilty as I knew that I had done everything I possibly could do and that we needed professional help.

At the end of June 2023, I was visiting Adrian four times a week. Some people asked me if I was visiting every day, and their questioning look could have made me feel guilty for not doing enough, but I had tried visiting that often and I nearly fell apart emotionally and physically. I started to feel guilty but then I felt angry that they seemed to be judging me. I had been there for my husband, putting much of my life on hold, visiting, loving, coping, despite how difficult it was at times. The care home staff encouraged me to go and enjoy myself, to enjoy my family, to go on holiday and to live my life while I was still able. They reassured me that Adrian was well looked after, that they loved him, and I was so grateful to the consistent staff team who understood and responded to Adrian's needs.

Earlier that month I had spent a week in Cornwall visiting my mum and my sister and her family. I justified going by saying that my family was important and that my mum was old, and she needed me to visit, but I could have just said I needed a break and I wanted to go. I enjoyed being able to have a week off from visiting, time by the sea, time with my family and going out for coffee and meals. I gave myself permission to meet my own needs and to enjoy life even if Adrian could not join me. Adrian's life seemed so limited, but he was happy in his own way. There were so many things he now couldn't do but he also had no desire to do them. One sunny day we managed to go for a little walk outside, a mammoth success, but he wanted to go back fairly quickly and sat peacefully in the lounge with the other residents where he felt safe and comfortable. I wanted more than that though, to live my life, to have a passion for life and to receive the abundant life that Jesus came to give us. I loved the verse found in the Bible, "I have come that they may have life, and have it to the full" (John 10:10). I realised, sadly, that I had to do that without Adrian, without feeling guilty. I had done so many things with Adrian, including travelling, and I still wanted him there with me but that was now not possible.

The fourth stage of grief is depression. I was not depressed in the clinical definition of depression, but my energy levels were depressed. I was surviving and even having periods of enjoyment but underneath there was a despair, a heaviness. During Covid there was a sense of surviving. As Covid restrictions eased at various times, I started using our house as a gathering place, as Adrian and I had planned. I threw myself into work at the Care Centre and I was ensuring that I did things for myself to keep myself healthy. Each activity, each experience had its own joys and satisfactions, but then when each had finished, I seemed to be drowning in a sea of despair. There were enough islands in this sea of despair to keep me going, enough good things for me to keep my head above the water, enough support, love and prayers to keep me lifted and afloat. I sometimes felt a passion for living my life, but I also wanted to curl up and hibernate. The passion came and then disappeared, depression and despair reappeared and even the anger melted away into nothingness.

Early on in my therapy, as Colin indicated in the foreword, my tie-dye leggings became a symbol of where I was emotionally. They had a blue background that represented the sea of despair but there were other colours that looked like islands: islands of hope and satisfaction. Each island had something positive but then I sank into the sea of despair. My life was not integrated, it was fragmented with two parts to it: my life with Adrian in the care home and my life outside the care home. I don't know if my determination to keep going was healthy or not, but I know that passivity would have brought me even lower, and I needed to have some kind of normality at least in some of my life. I needed a sense of control and purpose other than caring for Adrian. At times, though, I had to step back from activity and grieve real feelings.

Chapter 10

The Roller Coaster of Acceptance

The fifth stage of grief is acceptance. I had started to accept that Adrian was probably not going to be healed miraculously but then he started to improve again. "He's getting better," I cried as I saw a change in Adrian. He was settled, seemed less anxious, happier and much less agitated. He started telling me more often that he loved me. He was not frightened anymore and was, on many occasions, happy to go outside in the garden and to even walk down the road a bit. The staff were thrilled as he started eating more, putting on much-needed weight, talking more and telling them when he needed the toilet or changing. One day he didn't want me to feed him and took the spoon and fed himself. He started asking questions.

"Where am I?"

"Are you OK?"

"What am I meant to be doing?"

I was not imagining it. The staff said the same.

"He's getting better."

"He greeted me in the morning."

"He's getting a personality."

"He talked to me."

"He smiled and laughed."

"He joined in."

I wondered what had led to the change. Maybe he was just more settled, and we could enjoy being in the lounge together, sitting on a settee together, having a cuddle and even a kiss, rather than being confined to his room as in the Covid days. He often smiled when I arrived saying, "Lovely," in greeting and appeared pleased to see me. He started being assertive about what he wanted, even saying, "Let's go back now," when we had been outside, communicating his wishes when he didn't want to do something or if he wanted to go somewhere else. He even started answering my questions. I believed God was starting a healing process and all thoughts of getting on with my life disappeared into a determination to visit more frequently.

But then there were the days when he was not so alert, and I questioned whether he was really getting better or was I seeing the good days and then the bad days, which the staff had warned me about. Sometimes he seemed to understand what I was talking about and other times I didn't know what he understood. Sometimes there was a real connection and we had beautiful eye contact with an obvious love still there between us. One day I was cuddling up to him and praying a heartfelt powerful prayer. When I looked at his face he was beaming, and he looked like he had really experienced the Holy Spirit. On some days I yearned for him to put his arms around me, to instigate a hug or a kiss. I sometimes felt abandoned by him and willed him to say that he loved me. The times he looked at me with such love and told me, "You're beautiful. I love you" made my day. When he reached out to hold my hand it meant so much, yet it was so far from what we used to have.

One day in early October 2022 Adrian was in bed. He had a bad cold and a chest infection. He had been taking antibiotics for a few days and was on the mend. He was tired, though, and the staff had put him to bed in the afternoon. I arrived at 4:15pm. He was sleeping so I just sat next to him and prayed. I sensed God in the room with us. There was a peace, and I felt the presence of the Holy Spirit and angels. Eventually Adrian awoke and smiled at me. We held hands and I started singing softly, worship songs that were full of love and peace. Adrian was mesmerised and we locked eyes as we felt such love for each other and from God. Adrian repeatedly whispered "lovely" and "wonderful". I don't think we had ever before spent so much time having such wonderful eye contact. The atmosphere in the room was tangible, full of love and peace and well-being. Songs were coming from me that I didn't know, songs of worship to a loving God. I could sense that Adrian felt what I was feeling, and we both were transported to a place of love and peace. I stopped singing and Adrian spoke, "You're lovely. I love you," and kissed me on the lips.

That experience was so precious to me as we spoke out our love for each other, with our eyes, our hands and our lips. Dementia had not robbed us of a loving relationship, had not robbed us of a sense of God's presence, had not robbed us of a tangible togetherness.

Two weeks later, though, I was back to concern and a sense of helplessness. I was aware that Adrian had been ill and had antibiotics, and on top of that he had had a flu and Covid vaccine, but he also seemed to be declining and spending so much time asleep in bed. I tried to find out if there was something bothering him. When he briefly touched his head, I wondered if he had a headache. His gums looked sore, so I feared toothache, but he was unable to tell me if anything was hurting him. He could not walk alone without losing his balance, so the carers did not want him out of bed. He had always been an active person, even with dementia, but now he was weak and bedridden for most of the day. I had seen other residents lying in bed in their rooms and I wanted to scream at Adrian to not get like them, to try hard and to not give up. They sometimes didn't even look alive and then they were not there, hopefully gone to a better place. I urged God to heal Adrian but if he would not, then take him before he was totally incapacitated. I didn't want to face this journey, but I still wanted to be there for him, wherever the journey took us, so I decided to get into bed with him. It felt normal to cuddle up with him and we started to hug and kiss and to feel the love we still had for each other.

That day when I went home, I tried to process what was happening. I questioned whether God had really told me and others that he would heal Adrian. I faced the fact that when the first symptoms of dementia appeared, Adrian was a young and vibrant sixty-seven-year-old, but now he was seventy-three and getting frail. Maybe now he was heading towards the inevitable death that we all have to face. He was no more special than the many others bedridden with this awful disease, when the brain does not remember how to tell the body to work. I hated the long haul of dementia, the years of decline, with the good and bad days, but I wanted to make the best of the days ahead and appreciate that we still had a closeness despite the awfulness of it all. I would keep the promise I made, in sickness and in health, not because of a ceremony but because of love.

November 2022 neared the end, but despite my fears of deterioration, Adrian had bounced back and seemed better and happier. He started talking again, even in whole sentences although some of the words didn't make sense. He liked looking at photos of us and when I told him about things we had done together he seemed interested. I was thrilled when one day he looked at me and said, "You are the most important person in my life for me"!

I was thrilled but so tired: tired with the emotional roller coaster, tired by using so much energy in encouraging him to talk and to understand, tired also with going more frequently. I wasn't sure whether I should go so often but as the staff were putting Adrian to bed more to stop him falling, I felt the pressure to go and walk with him or even sit with him. I felt the pressure to keep talking and encouraging him to talk, to pray and to build on our connection. I loved it when he was so pleased to see me, when we got into bed together and I could stroke his face and kiss his neck. I wanted him, though, to hold me and to touch me. I was grateful that he could receive but I wanted him to give too. Yet he gave more than was ever expected of him at this stage in the dementia. On one occasion he looked around and saw the pictures on his wall and he said, "I like it here." That was such a relief to me. He continued, "The people are nice."

Then the disappointment again as I was told that he kept banging at night and they were having to give him lorazepam as he seemed distressed. They also talked about giving him more olanzapine. I trusted the staff, but I felt so disappointed. It was such a roller coaster and so tiring! "God knows it is a roller coaster," said my friend Nicki, "but he says you are strapped in and safe." That made so much sense; God knew and understood and was there with me, ensuring I didn't fall. But where was this roller coaster taking us next?

The roller coaster continued for the next few months, times of excitement followed by times of disappointment and agony; times when there was a connection and then times when visiting seemed so pointless. The positive days included going down in the lift in a wheelchair and drinking hot chocolate, holding hands, having a meaningful conversation even in single words or phrases; times when we knew the love we had for each other. The negative days were just that: nothingness.

I was still seeing Colin, my therapist, who helped enormously especially with my confused feelings, which were sometimes bottled up and sometimes overwhelming. My feelings went up and down depending on how my visits with Adrian went. My life seemed to be just revolving around how he was, and the rest of my life had been put on hold. Colin encouraged me, though, to see my life as more than this, that my life also existed outside the nursing home, that I was still alive and I needed to live my life, that it didn't have to be put on hold.

One of the things that I had to come to terms with was the vision I had about using my house as a place of healing and refuge. I always thought it was our vision, our ministry together. Over the previous year I had sought to put that into practice. I had two retreat days for our church connect group, informal "bring your own" lunches after church, neighbours coming round for drinks in the new year and even friends living with me for six months while their new house was being built. I used the house for connect groups and for prayer times as well as friends gathering together. I was still keeping our vision alive, but I needed to own it as my vision. In some ways it seemed like a step backwards but in fact it was a step forwards towards accepting that Adrian was not part of the vision and did not even understand the vision, let alone be able to contribute to it. It was the beginning of doubting that God would heal him.

I talked to myself, reassuring myself that Adrian was peaceful, happy and well-cared for. I told myself he was OK, and that God was with him, but my heart broke as I questioned why God sometimes healed and sometimes he didn't. It was certainly not that I lacked faith. I had recently prayed for a lady who couldn't move her fingers and her hand was immediately healed, the pain and stiffness went, and she was instantly able to wiggle her fingers. Another lady was healed of a painful, ongoing back injury. I and so many others prayed often for Adrian, and I believed God had provided for him and he was happy, well looked after and peaceful, but the dementia remained.

Six years is a long time, nearly seven in fact. When he was sixty-seven I thought he was too young to have dementia, especially as he was so vibrant and energetic. But by this time he had reached seventy-four. Maybe I just needed to accept that he was over the "three score years and ten". We had such plans but now his age had caught up with him and it was not just the dementia affecting him. He seemed so much younger than the others in the care home when he first arrived but now he was weak and more fragile than he used to be. I started to think I just needed to rejoice in the outstanding care he was getting, rejoice in the promised life after death with Jesus, rejoice in the special times when we connected, and we knew that we loved one another and knew that we would be together in the next life.

There were times when I praised God for providing such excellent care for Adrian, times when I also enjoyed my life away from the care home. I remember one day when I spent the journey to Adrian's care home praising God, telling him I loved him, singing in the Spirit with words that were beautiful to hear, and I arrived feeling optimistic. Two of the carers who were always so welcoming greeted me, saying they had just changed Adrian, that he had eaten and drunk well and that he was ready for us to have an enjoyable time together.

When I saw him, he reached out his hand to me, let me kiss him and then pushed me away. Then he seemed to zone out and from then on didn't acknowledge me. We had been here before when I had sat and waited, prayed and stroked his arm or held his hand, sometimes massaging his feet whilst he slept or disappeared somewhere inside himself. That day, though, I couldn't do it. I wanted to wail and scream. I looked at Adrian, hoping he would see my distress and come back to me, but he didn't, so I just stormed out, got into my car and told God I hated him.

You may think I was risking it telling God I hated him, but I didn't care. I didn't care about anything. I just wanted to escape. I thought, "Maybe I will stop going to see Adrian, but I won't. Maybe I won't cope but I will. Maybe I will stop loving God, but I will still love him." I felt so mixed up. I questioned God, "What reason do you have for allowing dementia, the slow decline, the bereavement that goes on and on, the grief with no let-up, no sign of ending, just day after day after day of cognitive decline and helplessness?" God seemed to understand I just needed a break and in April 2023 I went on a Norwegian cruise with my daughter Lisa, her husband Neil and my two grandsons George (aged sixteen) and Ryan (thirteen). Colin was right, I needed to live my life and meet my needs, to know that I was important, that I could enjoy my life and have fun. I had a wonderful time enjoying the scenery, the family time, the food, the drinks, the entertainment, the break from home and the weariness I was feeling. We were there for one week. I could have managed two very easily.

The break had given me time to recuperate and also to think more clearly.

I wrote the following in my journal:

> One of the things I have realised is that Adrian's life is his and mine is mine. I cannot live his life for him. I cannot be there all the time and in fact it is not necessary. He still has a strength, a faith, a spiritual awareness and even relationships away from me. He is not depending on me. It is important that I go to visit him as I do make a difference, but he has a life other than with me. He may need a lot of help, practical help, but he is not helpless. There are times when the carers tell me that he has been talking or laughing. He has a relationship with them. There are times when he seems to be experiencing a peace that has nothing to do with me as though he is aware of a spiritual reality whether I am there or not. He has always been strong and resilient and that has not gone away even if he needs 24-hour care. He is still determined at times even if it is to say "no" to a particular food or drink or when he is insistent that he feeds himself when the carers are trying to help him. There is still an inner strength

even though now he needs help with walking. I feel so sad that he is losing his mobility, but he hasn't lost himself.

Adrian has always loved people and being with people. The carers love him and see beyond the practical help they are giving to the inner person who is still there. They tell me he is a kind man, a lovely man, a gentle man, a good man. They talk of his gratitude when they help him. They talk of smiles and laughter, of peacefulness and relationships. They say he is happy. They know what he likes and doesn't like. They want to make a difference and they do.

I cannot live his life for him. I can love him and keep visiting but he has a life away from me. That is so hard to accept but also so freeing.

I also have a life to live. It is my life. I am alive and I need to live the life that I have been given. Adrian and I have always been close, real, loving and authentic but we also had our own careers, our own friends, our own interests and activities. It is actually no different now. This is freeing. I am not only allowed to live my life, it is necessary and important to do so. It can be so difficult when those you love are in need of care, to continue with those interests and activities. There is a sense of guilt if I enjoy when he is unable to. There is sorrow and sadness that he is spending his days in a care home while I am seeing the world, and yet he is happy, settled and loved. I cannot make it any better by not enjoying myself.

I am so grateful for the relationships Adrian has with the staff. I am so grateful to them that they see beyond the practical help they give and see the person inside. I am really astounded that they are so loving. Yet they are also responding to him and his love for them. He often says "lovely" when they do something for him, when they give him a cup of tea or biscuits. The other day he said "lovely" when he was being given a shower. He enjoyed the water running over his face. That is healing! Before he was sectioned, he would not go near water for a fortnight and refused to wash. He enjoys being in bed and resting and sleeping. Yesterday when I arrived, he was in bed just smiling to himself. Who am I to say he is not enjoying his life? Sometimes I think he is aware of angels in his room. There is a sense of peace in his room that I believe is God. Sometimes other residents come and sit in there. They seem to feel the peace.

Yesterday one resident, I will call him Gary, walked in. Gary gets very confused and agitated. He knows we pray. He walked in and said, "Can you pray a blessing on me? I can't cope. I need Jesus." Another lady, we'll call her Mary, followed behind, sat down and wanted me to pray for her too. Then a carer came in with a milkshake for Adrian and started talking about life and life after death. She was wondering what was beyond this life, talking about spirituality and faith and saying she is exploring what she believes. Adrian still has a ministry to people. We still have a ministry together. It is not what we planned but I need to see his life from a different perspective. I remember back to what I said many years ago that I believed that even if someone was cognitively impaired, they can enjoy life if they are loved and not in pain. I am seeing that now. I believe it even though it is tough to watch the decline of someone I love. Is the life that others are living in this world any better than Adrian's life? Is running in the rat race, the chasing after fame, power and riches or wars, abuse and oppression any better than the love that Adrian has in his life? An emphatic no!

I also want that life, a life of love, of living the abundant life that God promises (John 10:10).

Then Adrian developed a persistent cough, and I was warned that he could choke on his phlegm when the staff were not with him. I was told that he might not die for years but it could happen at any time as his swallowing reflex was not good. His drinks now had to be thickened so that he could manage swallowing better and so he would not get liquid in his lungs. I started thinking about Adrian's funeral, which made me feel awful. As part of my attempt to live my life and to do something for myself, I had started guitar and piano lessons and was learning how to play one of Adrian's favourite songs, "Oceans" by Hillsong, and imagined it being sung at his funeral.

"Oceans"

You call me out upon the waters
The great unknown where feet may fail
And there I find you in the mystery
In oceans deep
My faith will stand

And I will call upon your name
And keep my eyes above the waves
When oceans rise
My soul will rest in your embrace
For I am yours and you are mine

Your grace abounds in deepest waters
Your sovereign hand
Will be my guide
Where feet may fail and fear surrounds me
You've never failed and you won't start now

So I will call upon your name
And keep my eyes above the waves
When oceans rise
My soul will rest in your embrace
For I am yours and you are mine

Spirit lead me where my trust is without borders
Let me walk upon the waters
Wherever you would call me
Take me deeper than my feet could ever wander
And my faith will be made stronger
In the presence of my Saviour[3]

---

3. © 2012 Hillsong Music Publishing (admin. Capitol CMG Publishing)

I was starting to accept that God might not have plans to heal him and might be taking him to be with him in heaven where he would have a new healthy body. I imagined him in green pastures with lush grass and beautiful flowers, sweet aromas and sunshine. It looked and smelled like paradise. In the picture I saw him waiting for me. Maybe healing was going to be in the next life.

The roller coaster continued, though, because as I contemplated Adrian's death, he bounced back. He was still very determined. I hadn't been with him at mealtimes for a while but one day I stayed for the evening dinner. Adrian was so determined to feed himself as much as he could and also decided what he would eat on his plate and when he would drink. It was a very slow process but his desire to be independent was amazing. In fact, his determination was incredible compared to a few months ago when he passively allowed others to feed him.

One of the carers often prayed for us both and Adrian always responded in some way, with a sense of peace or a smile or a nod. On that same day he seemed energised after prayer and got up out of his chair with no help and walked determinedly with some support for balance. One minute I was preparing for his funeral and the next I was rejoicing over improvement and small answers to prayer. He was generally less sleepy and more alert, talking again in single words or phrases. Every time I thought he was deteriorating he surprised me!

One thing I was very sure about was that spiritually he was not dying. Spiritually he was very much alive. There was a real anointing of the Holy Spirit that seemed to be increasing rather than declining. He was present spiritually even though his brain was not functioning well, and he still knew me and loved me. There was still eye contact and a connection between us. One of the carers told me that we had challenged her understanding of dementia, as in the many years she had worked in the field she had never seen someone with such advanced dementia maintain a relationship like the one we had.

I often had pictures of my journey, sometimes I had dreams of being in trains or cars or planes, where I had no idea where I was going. Some of these pictures and dreams seemed significant and stayed with me. Colin and I explored them to see what I was feeling and experiencing.

One such picture was of me climbing a steep mountain. The mountain was named dementia and I wanted to reach the top. I am not sure what I expected at the top, maybe to overcome dementia and reach the healing I was expecting for Adrian. In the picture I was halfway up and feeling stuck. I stopped on a ledge and could not see a way up or down. I looked out into the distance and I saw my past life with all I had achieved and experienced. I was amazed and encouraged by all I could see but it also seemed as if that life was over. I was stuck on the mountain of dementia. I had activities in my life, but my heart was on this ledge, stuck with nowhere to go. In the picture I heard a voice telling me to look behind me. I realised I was in front of a cave, and I could see that at the rear of the cave was a tunnel. The voice said it was the tunnel of acceptance and that I needed to stop struggling up the mountain and to walk through the tunnel of acceptance. On the other side of the mountain I would find a new freedom. In my mind's eye I could see a vast, lush meadow filled with buttercups. I saw myself dancing barefoot in the meadow. It was so spacious and beautiful. My life would continue and there would be joy but to get there I needed to go through the tunnel of acceptance. I was scared of the tunnel but in fact it was flat, wide and clear. I had to make a decision to stop fighting and struggling and accept that whatever I did I could not cure dementia. I had to let go and give Adrian back to himself and to God.

Another picture I had was of me desperately trying to swim upstream. I was met with a boulder in the way. I was struggling and trying hard. After a powerful therapy session, I realised that I needed to let go and to flow with the river, flow with life and with the Holy Spirit. I had always tried hard, even my school reports all seemed to include "Susan tries hard". There is a time to try hard but there is also a time to flow, to just live and not to control or over-plan. There was such freedom as I allowed myself to flow and to trust myself, life and God.

I expressed this in my journal:

I have decided to live, not just to survive. It feels like water flowing – fast, slowly, round bends, over stones, deep, shallow, over waterfalls. It's not a struggle – water doesn't have to try or work hard.

It goes with the flow. I don't have to struggle or work hard. Sometimes it might feel rocky or scary, sometimes restful, sometimes round bends not knowing where it's going next, sometimes energetic and sometimes languid. It doesn't plan. I over-plan when I get scared, stressed or anxious.

At church on Sunday, I started moving to the music and I felt like I was flowing, like life flowing through me and I felt a lightness.

Living means feeling the feelings, including painful ones, but also having fun and being spontaneous and free. It reminds me of being with Adrian before he became ill. He helped me to live and feel. I don't want to lose what he gave me but now I have to make that life my own without his support. It's like riding a bike without the stabilisers.

Chapter 11

Aspiration Pneumonia

One morning at the end of April 2023, I got a phone call from the care home telling me that they had phoned 999 as Adrian was in distress and couldn't breathe properly. He was coughing so much that he could not catch his breath. Quickly, I donned some clothes. I wanted to pray as I drove, but I sensed God saying to me, just drive and concentrate. I realised this was pretty important, especially in my panic.

When I got to the home, the paramedics were there. They were so professional, kind and caring, and they were not panicking. They had aspirated Adrian and given him oxygen and had just transferred him to a trolley to take him to hospital. I left my car and sat in the ambulance, holding Adrian's hand. Many people complain about the care they get in hospital, but I was so grateful for all those who helped us: the A&E staff, then the Resus team and eventually the Acute Admissions ward.

In Resus, Adrian was wired up to monitors and a drip. Sometimes the monitors beeped, and my first reaction was that he was dying. I am sure there were angels in the room, and I sensed God's presence even in my anxious state. My prayer was, "Please, God, make him better or take him as I don't want him to suffer a long, difficult death. I would rather he went to paradise." It was awful hearing him cough so that he couldn't breathe properly. The nurse looking after him, though, was calm and aspirated him, giving him relief.

Many people were praying, and I am so thankful for all the love and support. I am also grateful to have a smartphone so I could be in contact with my family, friends and church.

I stayed with Adrian all day, holding his hand, praying, just being there. I wanted to be his voice, to make sure his needs were being met. I was afraid to leave him, in case the staff didn't understand how bad his dementia was. They were very patient with me and reassuring so that when my son Geoff came to pick me up, I knew I could leave Adrian safely in their hands. The care home staff were brilliant, ensuring that the hospital was aware of all Adrian's needs. Maybe I should have been more trusting and not thought I was the only one who could be Adrian's advocate! In fact, some of the questions I was asked, I didn't know the answer to and had to refer the ward staff back to the care home. I could also trust God and, in fact, Adrian himself who seemed peaceful when I left.

As I was picking my car up from the care home, I went in to get some clean clothes for Adrian and to talk to the staff. They were all very caring but also a bit frightening as they were talking about the fact that Adrian was even choking on his own saliva and that we needed to put plans in place when he came back to the home. Last stage dementia was mentioned, and palliative care was implied.

"God, please help us!"

Adrian was transferred to a ward, and I visited daily. I don't think I realised before how tiring it is just sitting next to someone's hospital bed. It was emotionally draining, especially after the shock of the emergency admission. When he first went to the care home I was asked where I would want him to be, hospital or care home, if he needed palliative care. It was a question I didn't even want to consider at the time but now the question had arisen again.

I was still amazed at the peace Adrian felt even in hospital in a strange ward with staff he did not know. I remembered back to the fearful, anxious man who was paranoid and psychotic, and I marvelled at how much he had changed. His mental health was so stable, and he was eating and drinking well. The SALT (speech and language therapist) put him on a pureed diet and thicker drinks and Adrian managed well on them. He was also grateful to the nursing staff, saying thank you to them. One nurse who I had never met before, came into the bay, looked at Adrian and told me, "He is a good man." I was proud of Adrian but also a bit surprised that the nurse could see who Adrian was when he was so unwell. God was still shining out of him. As I wrote before, "Oceans" was a song that Adrian loved, and I sang it to him a few times as he was lying in the hospital bed. The man in the next bed spoke to me. "Thank you for singing," he said. Then he started crying so I went over to him. "It's the love," he said. "It's the first love I have felt for several weeks." I held his hand, talked with him and then prayed for him. He felt the peace and love of God and proclaimed that he thought he could sleep now. Adrian and I still had a ministry to hurting people who were craving for love.

The doctors on the ward were very attentive to Adrian. The consultant had wondered whether Adrian was on too much olanzapine, saying that he was not psychotic or agitated so maybe he didn't need the medication, and, as it had a sedative effect, it could have caused some of his drowsiness. He suggested that Adrian's swallowing could be affected because he was too drowsy, and that food and drink went into his lungs causing the aspirational pneumonia. If he was less sedated maybe he would swallow better. As Adrian was still on antibiotics the consultant delayed starting the reduction but would start a behaviour chart identifying a baseline so that they could compare when he was on less medication.

Going back to the question of where I wanted Adrian to spend his last days, I had eventually stated that I wanted him in the care home where he knew the staff so that he would not be confused or agitated, but now I was not so sure. There were constant attentive staff in the six-bedded bay he was in, and the doctors were on hand. The care home relied on the local GP usually by phone or video link. Adrian was really settled in the hospital and had the medical care he needed, so I prayed that he didn't go back to the home until the right time.

I found it so difficult. I loved my husband so much, but I didn't know what I wanted for him anymore. Some people would be shocked that sometimes I just wanted him to die and to go to heaven. I told him that Jesus had prepared a place for us where we would be together with him. I told him if he wanted to go first that he could go, and I would catch him up. I didn't know what he understood. Sometimes he seemed to understand, yet other times I knew he didn't, like the time the nurse asked him to lift up his arm so she could take his blood pressure. I had to explain that he didn't understand and then I helped him to comply.

When I first believed Adrian would be healed, I imagined him coming home. I confess by this time I couldn't contemplate what that would look like. I couldn't see how it would work. I thought about what would happen if he was partially healed. I really didn't want to face being his carer at home even if he was calm and peaceful. I couldn't envisage the continued journey. I couldn't imagine a miracle in the way I first believed. I wanted others to care for him and maybe selfishly I wanted a life. I wanted to move on, not by abandoning him but by accepting this phase of the journey.

Nine days after his hospital admission the doctor told me that Adrian was ready to be discharged. I was so surprised as he was still coughing, not as badly as he had been, but the cough was still there. The doctor assured me that the infection was cleared up and then added that Adrian would still be coughing as he had a problem with swallowing. He explained that this would inevitably lead to further infections, and I would need to plan for end-of-life care. I had a choice as to whether he would go back into hospital for IV antibiotics, have oral antibiotics whilst remaining in the care home, or decide not to have any antibiotics. In my head I screamed that I didn't want that responsibility, I wanted more information, I needed advice, I needed support. I felt so shaky, and I felt such a heavy weight on my shoulders.

Many people caringly told me that I had to look after myself and in some ways I understood what they meant. They saw that I was tired after nine days of being with Adrian in hospital, of going through the crisis and caring for him. They recognised that I had given out and needed refreshing and building up again. They knew how much I loved and cared for Adrian, but they wanted to make sure I was not neglecting my own care. I had often said the same to others when they were going through similar demanding life experiences. I remembered many times saying it to my friend Nicki when she had a lot of significant family demands. It was a long time later that she said, "I don't really know what that means." I was feeling that now. Nicki and I both knew some of what it meant: eating healthy food, keeping hydrated, resting and doing something for ourselves. It sounded easy but much harder to do in practice.

Many people said that I needed to rest and not do too much, but resting was difficult, and I hated being bored. I didn't want to sit and watch daytime television.

Maybe, though, it meant doing what I enjoyed doing. I had planned to lead a training session and decided that I didn't want to cancel it. I became energised with the thought of doing something that I was enthusiastic about and was good at. It made me feel alive after so much sickness, treatments and even possible end-of-life care. Others noticed the difference in my demeanour, from the weariness beforehand to the alertness and enthusiasm throughout the evening. Maybe looking after ourselves is different for each of us. Maybe in the face of illness and decline in those we love, we need to look after ourselves by doing those things that make us feel alive. It can be extremely easy to feel guilty about getting on with our lives when our loved one is declining, but denying ourselves life is not helping them or us. In fact, looking after ourselves by living life could enhance our ability to keep going on the marathon that is dementia.

Adrian went back to the care home on a Friday. The staff were all pleased to see him, and they said that he seemed pleased to see them. I decided that I would go back to my plan of accepting that he had a life outside of our relationship and that I could trust him and the carers with his life. I gave myself permission to visit him every other day on average.

I spent Sunday with my daughter and family. It was so lovely being cooked for, talking, playing games and relaxing in her hot tub. I felt physically and emotionally refreshed. Then, on Monday, it was the Coronation bank holiday and I had planned a buffet lunch and afternoon in my home. It was a really enjoyable time with children playing, people chatting, eating and drinking. It was so lovely being with friends and family, and I realised how much I needed enjoyment and company. I also booked a hair appointment and time to get my brows waxed and tinted. I needed things to build me up again after the stress of the previous weeks.

Adrian had been back in the care home for four days. I had visited twice and talked at length to the nurse there. I was trusting the staff to do the best for Adrian. Then I got a phone call telling me that Adrian was coughing and very distressed with an elevated temperature and fast pulse. The ambulance had been called, although this time it was not an emergency so I said I would meet them at the hospital.

I spent the day with Adrian and left when they had found him a bed in AAU, and I had reassured myself that the nurses knew about Adrian's dementia and his needs. I got home exhausted and with so many questions and concerns. The next morning I cancelled my appointments and went back into carer mode.

Chapter 12

What Love!

Jesus said, "By this everyone will know that you are my disciples, if you love one another" (John 13:35).

I was told I had to wait until visiting time to see Adrian, so I popped into Vineyard (my church) before going to see him. I was met with such love. So many people hugged me with such feeling, not just a quick hug but a bear hug of love that felt so real and authentic. They could not provide a quick fix, they didn't even offer to say a prayer with me, they just loved me. They knew my pain and they entered into it with me. Jesus said that his family were those who followed him, who believed in him and at that moment I was so grateful to belong to such a loving family. We often want to make everything better, to fix a difficult situation, to get rid of the pain, but what might be needed is to stay in the pain with a hurting person. At the hospital I was asked if I lived on my own and whether I had support. Although I lived on my own, I did not feel alone.

I am not saying that prayer is a bad thing. These people had prayed, they were still praying, they would continue to pray, but saying a prayer can be a way to distance ourselves from the other person's pain, a quick fix to protect us from feeling the pain and entering into it. Just loving me, physically loving me, helped me to feel less alone. We missed so much of that in the pandemic when touch was not allowed. I am so pleased that I go to church where love can be freely expressed and where pain is validated and acknowledged, where we can be real and authentic, where we can acknowledge that life sucks sometimes.

Adrian was admitted to hospital, this time in an elderly care ward. I managed to negotiate getting in to see the consultant during the ward round despite the receptionist's best effort to stop me. Sometimes being politely assertive is important. Adrian could not answer for himself, and I needed to be his advocate, especially when I realised that important information had not been passed on from his previous admission. The consultant fortunately was glad I was there and in fact had caught up with the notes. He said that Adrian had had several bouts of aspiration pneumonia and was very poorly. I was shocked when he suggested that to stop this happening again there was a possibility of tube feeding him directly into the stomach. "But one of his pleasures is eating and drinking," I exclaimed. On reflection, that was not in fact true. I realised he loved the taste of food and drink, but he often gave up after a few mouthfuls. I was assured that he could have the experience of tasting food whilst being tube fed. After the initial shock, I warmed to the idea. The consultant explained that Adrian would get better nutrition and larger quantities, which would enable him to put on much-needed weight, he would become healthier, would be less likely to need antibiotics and would be able to have a better quality of life. I saw this as positive and started sharing this possibility with my friends and family.

I continued my daily hospital visits. Adrian was peaceful but very sleepy. He looked thinner and weaker, and I started thinking this was the beginning of the end. I prayed, "God, heal him or take him."

Six days after his admission, whilst waiting for the final decision about tube feeding, I was told he was ready to be discharged. My surprised questioning was answered with, "No, he isn't on the list for getting a PEG (tube) fitted."

"But the consultant said ... I need to speak to a doctor," I pleaded. I spoke to a helpful doctor who was with the consultant at our initial consultation.

"Adrian has improved better and quicker than expected. No gastroenterologist would agree to fit a tube. He is ready to go back to the care home."

I was so relieved but then later I questioned it, realising that he might continue to aspirate food and drink into his lungs and get recurring infections. I wondered if they were just giving up on him.

After one week Adrian was back in the care home and I was exhausted. Sitting by someone's hospital bed was so tiring, feeling helpless was so debilitating, wanting answers and not getting them was so frustrating and annoying.

The care home staff were worried when they saw Adrian's deterioration. He had lost so much weight and looked old and haggard. They planned a conversation with the GP to make end-of-life plans in case of further deterioration. It hit me then: I didn't want to lose him. I really did know that heaven might be the best option, but I wanted him with me. I wanted to scream and scream and scream. I couldn't do this, I couldn't watch him go, I couldn't let him go. I still wanted healing, I still wanted him back, the healthy Adrian, the one who in other circumstances would be comforting me and supporting me, the one who understood how I was feeling and stood with me in my pain, the one who I loved, my soulmate. I was helpless with no choice. Life and death were out of my hands. I had told him that we would be together in heaven, and I believed it. But suddenly it hit me that we were not talking about a little trip somewhere; we were talking about dying. I knew we all had to die sometime but it suddenly felt so real, and I felt shaky at the thought. Dying was irreversible, I would lose him, and he would never be here with me again.

Four days later Adrian was happy, smiling, talking and eating. He was pleased to see me and again said wonderful things to me and kissed me. He didn't seem ill; he wasn't coughing but I was warned that choking could happen anytime, and the doctor had prescribed end-of-life drugs that may or may not be needed. I was really confused and wondered whether to continue to visit him every day in case he was about to die or maybe I should give myself a break sometimes in case this was not the emergency I was told it was.

Adrian was now bed bound and was fed in bed with pureed food. Even his thickened tea was given to him with a teaspoon by the staff, although sometimes he wanted to take the cup and drink independently. I felt so sad when he reached for his biscuits, which were now not allowed, wondering where they were. I hated taking this minor act of independence from him, but I knew the staff were just being careful of food and drink entering his lungs.

I hated this roller coaster of uncertainty. We had been through a crisis that could have led to death. When he came out of hospital the care staff acknowledged that he was likely to die and hugged me with tender compassion. The next day they were amazed and said he was a new person, or rather back to the person they had come to love. But I had been warned that he wasn't swallowing properly and could choke at any time. Food, drink and saliva could be sucked into the lungs at any time. I had prepared myself and acknowledged that death could be a release and a relief for him and that he would be well and happy in heaven. Now he was smiling at me and was saying something I couldn't quite hear. "It was a joke," he laughed. We looked at photos of us, which we both really enjoyed. He seemed to understand more again and was talking more. He was awake and enjoying our time together. I was thrilled but also so confused.

Two weeks passed and Adrian started sleeping a lot. One day I arrived and he had his eyes open but was just staring, seemingly oblivious to me being there. I was mortified, wondering if this was him totally disappearing and I started willing Adrian to die peacefully in his sleep, so we didn't have to go through this awful period. I was dreading it and I felt so sad, so incredibly sad, and very lost. I also felt exhausted. I had decided to visit Adrian every day except one day when I went out with my daughter for a mum and daughter shopping trip with coffee and lunch. It was lovely but I felt so tired. The next day I just couldn't face going to the care home, I had no emotional energy left.

I realised I had stayed in crisis mode but at that moment there was no crisis. The staff reassured me that Adrian was eating and drinking and that he was much better than when he came back from hospital. With dementia there are days that are better than others and times when the brain seems to temporarily shut down. I knew this but I was so tuned in to crisis mode that I saw it as a sign of the end. I felt like I had been pacing in the waiting room, putting my life on hold, just waiting for what seemed like the inevitable ending. Therapy helped me a lot and I would recommend anyone going through this awful journey to get professional help with a counsellor or therapist that you can be real with. Colin helped me realise that I didn't have to stay in the waiting room and that the care home staff would contact me if necessary. I could go back to enjoying my visits with Adrian, but I also could have days when I didn't go, and I could do other things. I needed to realise the real danger of burnout, so I went to see Adrian with a different mindset, not expecting a crisis but just to enjoy being with him. It worked! I stayed for nearly three hours because he was awake. We enjoyed just being together, touching, listening to music and occasionally speaking. Quality time was so much more important than quantity. The peace I felt giving up on the crisis mentality possibly helped both of us. I needed to look after myself for both our sakes if I wanted to be there when Adrian really needed me. I also needed to recognise and accept that my life was also important. My needs were important. I had forgotten this or ignored it. I was allowed to think about myself as well as Adrian. If you are reading this and are in this situation, then just know that you are important, and your needs are important. You can enjoy yourself without guilt. I know how hard that can be, but it is really important, even if it is just to keep healthy for your loved one.

A month later I needed to listen to my own advice! Months before Adrian got pneumonia I booked a ten-day cruise with my friend Delia. I struggled at the time to agree to be away for ten days in case Adrian felt abandoned but now I was even more concerned about going away. The holiday was in seven days' time.

The week before we had such an amazing time and Adrian yet again surprised the carers. He wanted to get out of bed, so we sat him in a chair. The carer placed a table in front of him and then his dinner on the table. She turned round to get herself a chair ready to feed him. She didn't get the opportunity, though, as Adrian had picked up the spoon and fed himself perfectly, eating most of his dinner totally independently. He neared the end, pushed his plate away and said very clearly, "I don't want any more." She was so surprised and repeatedly said, "I am speechless!" Adrian then wanted to stand up, and pushed himself with great determination, although he didn't quite make it. Instead, we helped him into a wheelchair, and I decided to take him into the garden. I told him we would get a cup of tea when we got back. Sometimes I felt that Adrian was zoned out and was unaware of what was going on. That day, though, was different. He looked around and questioned me. "What are we doing here?"

I told him I thought it would be nice to get some fresh air and sunshine.

"That's stupid," he replied.

"I thought we could go for a walk," I replied.

"Where?" he questioned.

I pointed to the garden path. "Over there," I told him.

"Silly," was his reply.

I was surprised but pleased that he had responded appropriately. He had looked around, decided he didn't want to be there, asked questions and responded! Instead, we went inside, had a cup of tea and sat in the lounge. He was happy and later told me how much he loved me.

Two days later we had such a lovely time with him kissing me and stroking my arms, neck and face in a way that he had not done for so long. There was such a tangible sense of love, desire and intimacy. I was ecstatic!

Despite having accepted the fact of his imminent death, I now started wondering yet again if God was healing him.

Then I got a phone call. Adrian was coughing and was back on oral antibiotics and the GP wanted to know what I wanted to do if the antibiotics didn't work. Luckily the nursing staff agreed with me that we didn't have to make a decision yet, and in fact the medication seemed to be working and he started sleeping peacefully with less coughing.

I was in a dilemma about the holiday and spent my therapy session thinking about the different possible scenarios and how I would feel. I wanted to go away and I didn't want to let Delia down, but I questioned how I would feel if Adrian died while I was away. I needed a holiday, but I couldn't think about my needs or wishes. I just wanted to do the right thing, but I didn't know what the right thing was. In fact, there did not seem to be a right thing and maybe in many circumstances there is no right decision. Adrian might have carried on living for months, years even, or just days. I realised how exhausted I was and how much I needed the break if I was going to reach the finishing line of this journey. I knew that when I was feeling emotionally energised, I could be there for Adrian. I could be proud of how much I had been there and not backed away from the pain, but I could have a life too. Unless there was a real emergency I was going on the cruise and would enjoy the life God had given me. I could trust God to be with Adrian and I could trust the staff too, as well as my son Geoff, who would also be available. I accepted that this holiday was God's gift to me.

Chapter 13

The End

I was so glad I went on the cruise in July as I really enjoyed it, had a much-needed break and Adrian was fine and well looked after. There were no more crises and life carried on much the same for the next three months.

October 2023 arrived, and I was hurting and in pain as Adrian had deteriorated and I didn't know if he recognised me. I now understood those people who didn't come back and visit. It was too painful. I also understood those people who said they were not coming to visit because they wanted to remember their loved one as they used to be. This journey had been so long. I remember times along the way when it was hard, times along the way when I had been given crumbs to keep me going, times when I could enjoy seeing the real person below the dementia. But now I hardly remembered the good times before dementia was first apparent. I remembered the journey of dementia, but I was forgetting when he was a vibrant, intelligent young man, my lover. I tried to dredge up those memories, making sure I could remember but they seemed so distant and faded.

I felt affirmed when the carers praised me for visiting so regularly. Others, they said, can't or won't come so often or not at all. They were shocked at how others left their loved ones at this difficult time. I now knew how hard it was to watch the decline. I now knew the pull to want to keep the good memories alive. I now knew the desire to run. I was not even sure if Adrian knew that I was there or even recognised my touch or my voice. He was sleeping such a lot but seemed peaceful and he was still eating and drinking, but I felt like I could have been just any person holding his hand, stroking his forehead, giving him drinks. I would keep going, though, because he might just know me and feel loved through my touch, my kisses and my prayers. He might still be there inside the seeming shell of his body, knowing me in some way.

On Saturday 14th October when I visited Adrian, he was awake in bed. Usually when he was awake he loved having a drink, but that afternoon was different. He wasn't drinking but he also didn't seem to be refusing the drink, he just didn't seem to respond, and his jaw was clenched. I told the carers, who assured me they would try later. The next day I had a message to phone the home. I was told he was not eating and drinking and they asked me to come in despite the fact it was evening when visitors normally went home. I got myself ready and went with trepidation. I was told that this would be the end, but I suggested we try again to give him a drink. They did but I could see they were right; he seemed unable to drink. The night staff told me to go home, get some rest and come back in the morning. They assured me that they would phone if Adrian deteriorated. My daughter Lisa was on standby. Unfortunately, my son Geoff was ill and was asked not to bring his flu-like germs into the care home. My friend Cecilia was also on hand.

The next day, a Monday, I spent an incredibly special day with Adrian. I can't describe the nine hours I was with him. There was such a closeness that I knew he felt as well and there was such a sense of God's presence, so much love. Adrian was not distressed even though he was unable to eat and drink. I asked again if we could try. The nurse was clear, however, saying that if we tried he would only choke. He was not able to swallow, and he wasn't even able to make saliva; he would choke to death and that would be awful for both him and me. They tenderly told me to let him die peacefully.

That time together was awesome. I prayed and sang and told Adrian about all the good things he had done in his life. I talked about our love, and I talked about God's love. I told him again that Jesus had prepared a place for us both in heaven, and that when Jesus called him, he should go. I told him I would miss him, but I would be alright, and I had lots of support. I thanked him for all he had done for me. I thanked him for how he helped me to blossom and how he never put me down but always encouraged me to be confident in myself. I thanked him that he had provided for me, the beautiful house and the money he left for me. I read his favourite passages in the Bible. We held hands and we snuggled up in bed. He seemed to appreciate the kisses. I told him how proud I was of him, the way he had helped me and so many others during his life. I told him how proud I was for the way he had been a light in the care home and how so many people had seen his love and gentleness. I told him how proud I was for how he managed the dementia. He stayed awake and seemed alert, even though he didn't seem to be able to open his mouth to speak. I was amazed at the strength I had. I knew it was God with me, the numerous prayers that were being prayed for us both and the determination to love to the end.

At 7pm I was told quite forcibly to go home as Adrian needed his rest and they wanted me to be refreshed for the next day. I appreciated someone telling me what to do.

I was surprised I slept until I was woken at 6:45am by a phone call asking me to come back in. Adrian was deteriorating, although I was told I didn't have to rush as it would probably be a few hours yet. "Take your time, have breakfast," the nurse said. There was no way I could eat anything; I felt so shaky and confused, I even found getting dressed a mammoth task. I phoned Lisa who assured me she would be coming but as it would take her two hours, she ordered me to get someone to take me and to stay with me. Again, I appreciated being told what to do. Cecilia was ready for my phone call. There was no way I could drive, and I was so grateful to her for driving me and staying with me and I appreciated her company. The day before I had appreciated being on my own with Adrian but that morning it was good to have Cecilia with me and to pray alongside one of the carers for Adrian.

Lisa was such a support when she arrived and stayed with me. It got to lunchtime and I realised we both needed to eat. The nurse said there was time for her to go and get some fish and chips, which we could eat in Adrian's room. Although I appreciated the support, I also appreciated that time on my own with Adrian. It felt like a very personal goodbye just between the two of us when I could be so honest about our love and relationship. He stayed awake, looking peaceful even though his breathing was laboured.

At 2pm we were told not to go anywhere as Adrian's oxygen levels were going down. He was given morphine in case he was in pain, although he didn't seem distressed. At this point all I could do was hold his hand, tell him I loved him and smooth his forehead. I also prayed for a peaceful passing. All through this time I felt God's presence. I also knew there was an angel in the room. I had often felt this angel standing watch at the bottom of the bed. I can't prove it; I never actually saw it with my physical eyes, but I had a sense of the size and position in the room.

Suddenly, after two days of not being able to open his mouth, Adrian's mouth opened twice. I was next to him on the bed and could only see him sideways. Lisa, though, was opposite him and could see his mouth clearly.

"He's just said goodbye," Lisa exclaimed. "He was definitely mouthing goodbye."

At that moment I felt his spirit rise towards the angel.

"He's gone," I pronounced.

I looked at his body, which moved. I assumed then I was wrong but within a second or two I realised, yes, he had gone; his body had just shut down and life had departed. Adrian had gone to be with his heavenly Father in paradise. He had gone peacefully without a struggle, without hesitating, without pain or breathlessness. He was ready to go, and he knew where he was going. His faith was alive to the very end.

Later, as I walked back into the room, I was aware that the angel I had sensed for the whole time Adrian was in the home had gone. I can't explain but my spiritual eyes knew.

Initially it was a relief that Adrian had gone so easily and quickly without extended suffering. I was grateful that he had not gone when he had pneumonia earlier in the year. Despite the fact that I had been told he would probably have repeated bouts of pneumonia, he had in fact had a clear chest for several months. He didn't gasp for breath or struggle; he just went peacefully, and I knew God was there.

I was shown so much love in the time afterwards and at his funeral. It was good to hear so many people talk about his life and how much he made a difference to so many people.

I had been grieving for so long before Adrian died, as he deteriorated, and I thought maybe I had done most of my grieving, but I was wrong. There was an emptiness. I missed him, missed the touching, the praying, the togetherness that we had even when his brain was shutting down. In fact, I had a whole new lap of the grief journey to face. I had said I had lots of support and that was true. There was a circle of people surrounding me and I was so appreciative, but I was still alone in the centre of the circle, without my partner, my soulmate, someone who I could do life with, live with, share myself with and be intimate with. I missed him.

Chapter 14

Life After Death

I was thrilled with the way Adrian died. It was also a relief to know that he was not suffering, and he was with his heavenly Father in heaven. I had no doubts about the goodness of whatever his experience would be in the afterlife. I knew he loved Jesus and Jesus loved him and that there would be something glorious ahead for him. I wanted to still do the best for Adrian and organised a dignified funeral that was honouring to him. I thought I had accepted that God hadn't healed Adrian but had taken him to a better place. I arranged a thanksgiving service in which we rejoiced over who Adrian was, the things he had achieved and the help he had given to so many people. It was a wonderful service, and I felt the love of so many towards him and also towards me.

The stages of grief, though, started to repeat themselves. Intellectually, I knew Adrian had died but my desire to still be there for him through all the arrangements I had to sort out softened the blow and I think this was a type of denial. My hope in the afterlife had prevented me from experiencing all of my loss.

Afterwards, however, I wailed like a wounded animal, not quiet sobbing but a loud wailing. Some of my friends prayed for God's comfort but I didn't want comfort; I wanted to express the grief I felt. I felt lost, battered and weary.

I thought I had accepted Adrian's death, so I was so surprised that I entered the angry stage again. I was furious, especially with God. I vehemently questioned God again about not healing Adrian and denying us the life and ministry I thought he had promised. Colin encouraged me to be real with my anger, which helped but I didn't really want to be angry with God and I tried to move onto the stage of acceptance. I sat like a sulky child moaning that I supposed I had to accept because I could not do anything about it. I felt helpless but I was also still very angry. Acceptance did not sound like a positive thing; it felt like a very passive place to be. Colin seemed to agree that this form of acceptance was indeed passive, but he suggested there was another form of acceptance called radical acceptance. I looked it up and it made me even more angry. I realised I didn't want to accept but I also hated being angry with God. I loved God and I wanted his comfort. I knew he was there with me and would never leave me, but I hated the conflict I had within me, questioning why God had allowed this awful journey through dementia, questioning his goodness and his plans, and I wanted answers.

God was gracious, though, and started explaining to me that he knew what was best for Adrian and I had to look at this journey as a journey of his life, not mine. He reminded me of the emotional struggles Adrian had throughout his childhood, how he had overcome so much of his brokenness and then lived his life using all his energy to empower and equip others to become the best version of who they were made to be. He had put his whole self into his work and had made such a difference to so many people. He had also lived his life to the full, travelling the world, giving television and radio interviews and speaking at conferences, as well as loving, dancing and praising God. Even though I was ready for a new season of ministry and had a vision for retirement, Adrian had used up his physical strength. He encouraged me and put his money into our home as he knew this venture was from God. He also loved me and wanted to support my dream, but it was not in fact something he wanted for himself. He had no more energy to start a new ministry, a new venture, and his body was declining. I had thought that at the age of sixty-seven he was young and vibrant but many of his organs were declining. My understanding was that dementia suddenly appeared and that if that was taken away then he would be energetic and healthy, but that was not the case. Adrian was ready to rest and be cared for away from the pressures of life in the fast lane. His mother had had many struggles and often found it difficult to care for him as a child. The attentive, loving and tender care Adrian received in the care home was a gift that he had lacked in his early life. Death comes to all of us, and this was the right time for Adrian. As I reflected on these truths, I realised that this was radical acceptance, and I was so grateful to God for explaining it to me.

Irvin Yalom, in his book Love's Executioner,[4] writes of the inevitability of death. He speaks of two delusions that we use to allay the fear of death. One is the belief in personal specialness and the other in an ultimate rescuer. My journey depicts both of these. I believed that God would heal Adrian despite the fact that so many other people were dying with dementia. My magical thinking of my childhood was coming into play as I imagined God rescuing Adrian using his mighty power, yet God knew that this was not the best way.

As I stopped being angry I was able to rejoice in the provision God gave us through this journey, how he never left us, how we felt his peace, the connection we had together, the caring staff, the support, the blessings along the way, and I realised the awesome love God had for us.

Five months after Adrian died, the journey continues and I wrote the following in my journal:

I can now go on with God, embracing life, enjoying my future, building on the love Adrian and I had, and trusting in a God who is wiser than me. I still mourn and grieve and struggle at times, but I can live, really live the gift that is life in abundance. I still need support and courage. Life still can be a roller coaster of good and bad days. I still am

---

4.   Irvin D. Yalom, *Love's Executioner and Other Tales of Psychotherapy* (Penguin, 2013).

unsure of what moving on in my life looks like. I still sometimes look at my leggings and see the sea of despair with islands of enjoyment dotted within it and I feel fragmented. There are also other patterns on my leggings, and in life itself, that are full of hope and joy and colour. There is a burst of colour that reminds me that I am alive, that I have a future and a hope.

David Kessler, who worked with Elisabeth Kübler-Ross on the five stages of grief, has added another stage, that of finding meaning after the loss of a loved one.[5] This is the continuing journey of my life, to find meaning, not in the death of my soulmate but finding meaning in my life, appreciating being alive, appreciating the colourful patterns of life and entering into a fullness of life, even the roller coaster of life.

I am embracing the vision that God gave me and continues to give me, using my experience to journey with others, broken people who want life and restoration. Through my own journey I have learned to be authentic and real with myself, others and God. I want to flow in the next season of my journey, to be the best version of myself and to live in authenticity. I want to live the promise that Jesus gave us:

"I have come that they may have life, and have it to the full." (John 10:10)

---

5. David Kessler, *Finding Meaning: The Sixth Stage of Grief* (Scribner, 2019).

Made in the USA
Middletown, DE
01 November 2024